Poetry, Therapy and Emotional Life

Diana Hedges

Forewords by
Gillie Bolton
and
Ted Bowman

Radcliffe Publishing
London • New York

Radcliffe Publishing Ltd
St Mark's House
Shepherdess Walk
London N1 7BQ
United Kingdom

www.radcliffehealth.com

British Library Cataloguing in Publication Data

A catalogue record for this book is available from the British Library.

ISBN 978 185775 860 3

Typeset by Phoenix Photosetting, Chatham, Kent, UK

For my daughters, Ruth and Annie

Contents

Forewords vii

Preface ix

About the author xi

About the contributors xii

Acknowledgements xiii

Permissions xiv

PART 1

CHAPTER 1
Poetry and therapy: a common pathway 3

CHAPTER 2
Transitions in life: early stages 15

CHAPTER 3
Transitions in life: later stages 27

CHAPTER 4
Spirituality, nature and religion 37

CHAPTER 5
Attachment and loss 51

CHAPTER 6
Loss and regeneration 63

CHAPTER 7
Journeys 73

PART 2
Introduction 85

CHAPTER 8
Poetry in individual counselling and therapy 87

CHAPTER 9
Running creative writing groups 97
Miriam Halahmy

CHAPTER 10
Poetry in healthcare settings   107

CHAPTER 11
Using poetry with young people: survive and shine!   121
Claire Williamson

CHAPTER 12
The art of memory: poetry and elderly people   133
Graham Hartill

CHAPTER 13
Poetry in counselling training   143

To conclude   153
Further reading   155
Index   159

Foreword

Sunlight's a thing that needs a window
before it enters a dark room.
Windows don't happen.
(RS Thomas)[1]

This book is a window. With lucid clarity it throws light on the power of poetry to enlighten, inform and heal. In both the reading and the writing, poetry can heal because it enables understanding: slow and steady insight, and epiphanic flashes of *aha*.

We don't see things as they are, we see them as we are
(Anais Nin)[2]

Poetry is both a window into our inner selves, and out into the natural, social, cultural, historical and political worlds. It not only enables a clearer view of our connectedness, but also practical access both inwards and outwards.

The therapeutic potential of the expressive and explorative power of words has probably always been exploited. Psychotherapy is a much used and respected *talking cure*; poetry and other literary forms offer a *reading* and a *writing cure*. With deep professional and personal understanding of both psychotherapy and literature, Diana enables the reader to grasp, value, and implement the relationship between psychotherapy and poetry reading. Guest chapter authors offer insight into the therapeutic value of writing.

For too long poetry has been cast as difficult, obscure, only for the clever and initiated. The ear with which we need to listen and the hand with which we need to write, however, is that of the child. Diana, in her clear engaging prose (an art in itself), teaches how to find and use that ear and hand.

Gillie Bolton
Author in Reflective and Therapeutic Writing
November 2012

1   Thomas RS (1986) *Poetry for Supper*. In: *Selected Poems*. Bloodaxe, Newcastle upon Tyne. p 53.
2   Nin A. *The Diary of Anais Nin 1939–44*. Harcourt Brace, New York.

Foreword

As I have grown older, I have become convinced that it is in life's crossroads or transitions – living and dying, sickness and health, youth to aging, grief to hope, caregiver to care-receiver, school to work, belief and doubt, or from innocence to loss of innocence – that one needs to slow down, look both ways and be alert. *Poetry, Therapy and Emotional Life* is a book of and about crossroads. Diana Hedges organizes this stimulating book using a personal and family development lens to discuss life transitions, she invites her readers to slow down and consider the crossroads of life through the use of poetry, fiction, memoir and psychological insights to guide one's reflection. I was reminded of the closing lines of a Marge Piercy poem, writing about one of her crossroads, but also the crossroads of others: *She must learn again to speak.*[1] Her words mirror the old adage that if something is unmentionable, it can also be unmanageable.

Pioneers in the use of stories, writing and literary resources for therapeutic work asserted that the effectiveness of bibliotherapy depends in the facilitator's ability to choose material that speak to the individual's needs and interests; to make accurate, empathic interpretations of the his/her responses; and, through literature and dialogue to draw out deeper self-understanding.[2] Diana Hedges demonstrates these abilities. Be prepared as you read to discover yourself in someone else's story; to find confirmation or inspiration; and to relax as she guides you in enriching your emotional life.

Ted Bowman
Grief and family educator, poet and former board member of the
National Association for Poetry Therapy
Adjunct Professor at the University of Minnesota
and the University of Saint Thomas
November 2012

1 McCarty Hynes A and Hynes-Berry M (1986 and 1994) *Bibliotherapy – the interactive process: a handbook*. Northstar Press: St Cloud MN, p.18.
2 Piercy M (1973) To be of use. In: *Unlearning not to Speak*. Doubleday: New York, p. 38.

Preface

'Poetry makes nothing happen' wrote W H Auden in 1939, and since then his words have been used to justify or contest various views on the power or effectiveness of poetry. His words are usually understood as a challenge to Yeats' views on the power of poetry as a *political* force, rather than as a judgement on its aesthetic value.

In this book I hope to demonstrate that poetry can make, if not everything happen, at least a great deal, and to show that it is a powerful medium in which to express complex feelings and ideas. I specifically attempt to explore the strong inter-relatedness between poetry and psychological ideas. Both areas seek to illuminate the 'human condition', explain and describe issues such as love and loss, spirituality and transitions in life. Counselling and psychotherapy base their approaches on various psychological theories but in their practice seek imaginative and creative ways to work with people experiencing emotional distress in their lives.

The book is written in two halves: the first looks at what poets, therapists and counsellors have to say about human experience, the dilemmas that confront us, the drives and needs which influence our behaviour; the second is more practical in that it describes how literature, in particular poetry, can be used in therapeutic work. This includes work in psychotherapy and counselling, but also the work that is now being done by writers who run creative writing groups. My own background is in counselling, so the ideas about using poetry in counselling, counselling training and healthcare settings come from my own practice. I am delighted to be able to include three chapters by writers who do not regard themselves as counsellors or therapists, but who run creative writing groups with a therapeutic aim. Their experience is in different areas from my own, so they give the book a wider perspective than it would otherwise have.

In addition to counsellors and therapists, I hope that the book will also appeal to professionals in the field of health and social care. Such people witness daily, through their clients and patients, situations of change, loss, emotional upheaval and remarkable courage. It is easy to become overwhelmed by the enormity of it all: I hope that the poetry in this book will rekindle a sense of enthusiasm as people recognise the creative component of their work and sometimes see a fresh perspective. In addition to their working lives, professionals are often confronting these same concerns in their personal lives.

For writers who are interested in developing their therapeutic skills, I hope that the first half of the book will offer some insight into psychotherapeutic approaches. Part 2 should provide some further ideas with which to work with groups. I also hope that the book will appeal to anyone who has a love of poetry and who enjoys writing as a means of self-expression.

When describing psychological theories I have tended to stick to the originators of the theories – Freud, Jung, Rogers, Berne, Perls and Ellis. This is because I wanted to show how they approached issues of human motivation, experience and neurosis. They were, on the whole, highly original thinkers, who forged new concepts. In every case their disciples have developed and modified their ideas, but the core remains intact: it is this kernel that I have tried to convey. One of the advantages of teaching on an integrative counselling course is the opportunity it gives to become familiar with a wide range of therapeutic models. It is this that has led to my conviction that all the approaches I have described here have something valuable to contribute.

Lastly, in an attempt to avoid constantly referring to 'him or her' or 'he or she', I have usually referred to the counsellor or therapist as 'she' and to the client as 'he'.

Diana Hedges
November 2012

About the author

Diana Hedges worked as a social worker in hospital and local authority settings before moving into a career in counselling. She completed her counselling training at the University of Manchester in 1996, and since then has worked in private practice and for employee assistance programmes. She is a lecturer on counselling courses at Oxford University Department of Continuing Education. She has also developed courses on the relationship between poetry and therapy, and has facilitated creative writing groups in mental health settings. Diana has had a lifetime love of literature, especially poetry, and in her thirties she completed a degree in humanities with the Open University. She is a registered practitioner with the British Association of Counselling and Psychotherapy.

About the contributors

Graham Hartill is a poet and workshop facilitator. He was co-founder of Lapidus, worked in the fields of mental health and disability and was *Lifelines* facilitator for the Ledbury Poetry Festival for 8 years, working with elderly people. He is now writer-in-residence at HMP and YOI Parc Bridgend, teaches on the master's degree course *Creative Writing for Therapeutic Purposes* for the Metanoia Institute and, with Victoria Field runs the popular *Creative Writing in Health and Social Care* course at Ty Newydd, the Writer's Centre for Wales.

Miriam Halahmy is an author and a poet. She has published a novel for adults, *Secret Territory* (Citron Press, 1999), two poetry collections and short fiction for children, teens and adults. Her cycle of three young adult novels, *Hidden, Illegal, Stuffed* are published by Meadowside books (2011/2013). Miriam runs creative writing workshops in Highgate and also for asylum seekers through English PEN. She is a regular guest author at writers' conferences and literary festivals. Miriam appraises manuscripts and mentors emerging writers. She was chair of Lapidus (creative writing and reading for well-being) 2003 – 2005 and is an active member of London Lapidus. Miriam reviews books and contributes articles to a range of publications. She enjoys social networking through Twitter, Facebook and a variety of blogs. www.miriamhalahmy.com

Claire Williamson holds an MA in Literary Studies and a Certificate in Counselling. She has had two volumes of poetry published, *French Connections* (Firewater Press) and *Blind Peeping* (POTA Press), and has toured her short stories with Words Allowed. Her most recent undertaking has been as a librettist for Welsh National Opera. Claire has worked for 'Poetry Can' and 'The Poetry Slam' since 1995, and she has worked in a variety of community settings, including schools, prisons, healthcare settings, centres for people with learning difficulties and addiction recovery trusts. She is currently working on her second novel and a new collection of poems entitled *Ride On*.

Acknowledgements

Many people have helped and encouraged me in the course of writing this book. In particular I would like to acknowledge invaluable help from Rose Flint and Dr Robin Philipp in suggesting material for inclusion in the book.

I would like to thank Pat Silver, Ruth Anderson and Dr Kieron Winn for their insightful comments on the text.

I am very grateful to those clients, trainees and members of writing groups who allowed their work to be reproduced.

Appreciative thanks, also, to Lorna and John Clarke, Brian Donaghy, Diana and Peter Gallie, Rosie Hill, Hilary and Chris Lloyd, Claire and Mike Pike, Pamela Murray, Pauline Power, Lois Roberts, Yvonne Schmid, Pat Silver, Daphne and Roger Symon and Sue Weaver.

Thank you to Miriam Rowland and Andrea Hargreaves for their resourceful administrative support.

Finally, I would like to thank my editors Maggie Pettifer and Gill Nineham for their support, enthusiasm and guidance.

Permissions

Thanks are due to the following organisations that have kindly given permission for reproduction of copyrighted material.

Although we have tried to trace and contact all copyright holders before publication, this has not been possible in every case. If notified, the publisher will be pleased to make any necessary arrangements at the earliest opportunity.

Fleur Adcock. *For Heidi with Blue Hair* from *Poems 1960–2000*. Published by Bloodaxe Books, 2000. Reprinted with permission.

WH Auden. *Stop all the Clocks. Song IX from 12 Songs*. Originally published by Faber and Faber. Copyright © 1936 by WH Auden. Reprinted by permission of Curtis Brown Ltd.

Wendell Berry. *The Peace of Wild Things* from *Collected Poems 1957–1982*. Copyright © 1985 by Wendell Berry. Reprinted by permission of North Point Press, a division of Farrar, Straus and Giroux, LLC.

Gwendolyn Brooks. *We Real Cool* from *Collected Poems*. Published by Harper Collins Ltd. Reprinted by consent of Brooks Permissions.

Raymond Carver. *Late Fragment* from *All of Us*. Published by Harvill Press. Reprinted by permission of the Random House Group Limited. 'Late Fragment' from *A New Path to the Waterfall*, copyright © 1989 by the Estate of Raymond Carver. Used by permission of Grove/Atlantic Inc. any third party use of this material, outside of this publication, is prohibited.

Charles Causley. *Eden Rock* from *Collected Poems 1951–1997*. Published by Macmillan. Reprinted with permission of David Higham Associates.

C Cavafy. *Ithaka* from *Echoes*. Translation by Gerard Casey (1990). Rigby and Lewis, Crawley. Copyright © Gerard Casey. Reproduced by kind permission of Louise de Bruin.

EE Cummings. *I Thank You God for Most This Amazing*. Copyright 1950, © 1978, 1991 by the Trustees for the EE Cummings Trust. Copyright © 1979 by George James Firmage, from *Complete Poems: 1904–1962* by EE Cummings, edited by George J Firmage. Used by permission of Liveright Publishing Corporation.

Maura Dooley. *What Every Woman Should Carry* from *Sound Barrier: Poems 1982–2002*. Published by Bloodaxe Books, 2002. Reprinted with permission.

Carol Ann Duffy. *The Darling Letters* from *The Other Country*. Copyright

Krishnamurti J. Extracts from *Education and the Significance of Life* (1953). Copyright © Krishnamurti Foundation of America.

Laurie Lee. *April Rise* from *Selected Poems*. Reprinted by permission of PFD on behalf of The Estate of Laurie Lee.

C Day Lewis. *Walking Away* from *The Complete Poems of C Day Lewis*. Published by Sinclair-Stevenson. Reprinted by permission of The Random House Group Ltd.

Carson McCullers. *The Member of the Wedding*. Published by Cresset Press. Reprinted by permission of the Random House Group Ltd. Excerpt from *The Member of the Wedding* by Carson McCullers. Copyright © 1946 by Carson McCullers, renewed by 1973 by Floria V Lasky, Executrix of the Estate of Carson McCullers. Used by permission of Houghton Mifflin Harcourt Publishing Company. All rights reserved.

Kona Macphee. *IVF* from *Tails*. Published by Bloodaxe Books, 2004. Reprinted with permission.

Adrian Mitchell. *Beattie is Three* from *Adrian Mitchell's Greatest Hits*. Bloodaxe Books Ltd. Reprinted by permission of United Agents (www.unitedagents. co.uk) on behalf of The Estate of Adrian Mitchell. Copyright © Adrian Mitchell 1991.

Blake Morrison. *And When Did You Last See Your Father?* Copyright © Blake Morrison. Published by Granta Books. Reprinted by permission of Granta Books. Reproduced from © Blake Morrison 1993 by permission of United Agents Ltd. (www.unitedagents.co.uk) on behalf of Blake Morrison.

Sharon Olds. *Her First Week*. From *The Wellspring*. Published by Jonathan Cape. Reprinted by permission of The Random House Group Ltd.

George Orwell. *Why I Write*. Copyright © George Orwell 1953. Reproduced by permission of AM Heath & Co Ltd on behalf of Bill Hamilton as the Literary Executor of the Estate of the late Sonia Brownell Orwell and Martin Secker & Warburg Ltd.

Vasko Popa. *Give Me Back My Rags*. *Vasko Popa Complete Poems 1953–1987* translated by Anne Pennington and Francis R Jones. Enlarged edition published by Anvil Press Poetry in 2011.

Sheenagh Pugh. *Sometimes* from *Selected Poems* (1990). Reprinted by permission of Seren.

Kathleen Raine. *I Had Meant to Write* from *The Collected Poems of Kathleen Raine*. Copyright © Golganooza Press (2000). Reprinted with permission.

Siegfried Sassoon. *Everyone Sang* from *Selected Poems of Siegfried Sassoon* by Siegfried Sassoon, Copyright 1918, 1920 by EP Dutton. Copyright 1936, 1946, 1947, 1948 by Siegfried Sassoon. Reprinted by permission of George Sassoon and Barbara Levy Literary Agency and by permission of Viking Penguin, a division of Penguin Group (USA) Inc.

Dylan Thomas. *Fern Hill* from *The Collected Poems*. Reprinted by permission of David Higham Associates and *The Poems of Dylan Thomas* © by the Trustees

PART I

CHAPTER I

Poetry and therapy: a common pathway

When, during the celebration of his 70th birthday, one of his disciples hailed Freud as 'the discoverer of the unconscious,' he answered, 'The poets and philosophers before me discovered the unconscious. What I discovered was the scientific method by which the unconscious can be studied.'[1]
(Al Alvarez)

What is it about poetry that is therapeutic: that by reading or hearing a poem we can feel more alive, calmer, understood, energised, amused or wiser? How is it that poetry can validate our experience as well as enabling us to look at something in a fresh or different way? This first chapter explores these issues and also looks at some of the similarities between reading and writing poetry and the process of psychotherapy.

Effective poetry usually works on two levels: there is the content or idea of the poem and then *how* it is expressed – the language, imagery, rhyme and rhythm. The same is often true of therapy and other contacts between a client or patient and a professional. There is the 'issue', the content of the problem, but there are subtle ways in which communication is formed and maintained and experienced between the person offering help and the one seeking it.

Communicating strong feelings

It would be hard to imagine a single feeling that has not been expressed in a poem. Love, loss, anguish, joy, betrayal, excitement, disappointment, scorn, fear and anxiety are the stuff of poetry. This can connect us with our own strong emotions, but can also help to break down feelings of alienation and isolation. Others have experienced the same feelings. Elizabeth Drew (1959) describes it in this way:

> We read poetry because the poets, like ourselves, have been haunted by the inescapable tyranny of time and death; have suffered the pain of loss, and the more wearing, continuous pain of frustration and failure; and have had moods of unlooked for release and peace. They have known and watched in themselves and others.[2]

Poetry, then, can give us a sense of identity with the mood or thoughts or feelings of the poet. In addition, it broadens out our experience and helps us understand that some experiences, such as loss or making difficult moral choices, are not unique to us but are part of the human condition.

It can feel helpful to have a sad, distressed or troubled mood validated, but poetry also expresses affirmation and inspiration and offers hope. Lines such as:

I will arise and go now, and go to Innisfree
(William Butler Yeats, *The Lake Isle of Innisfree*, 1893)

Do not go gentle into that good night
(Dylan Thomas, *Do Not Go Gentle into that Good Night*, 1952)

Glory be to God for dappled things
(Gerard Manley Hopkins, *Pied Beauty*, 1877)

convey a feeling of energy and of action that is important for a sense of well-being.

Psychological insight

Poetry is not just an outpouring of emotion. Many poems explore complex patterns of thoughts or show how the poet moved from one thought through to another and either arrived at some conclusion or realised that he could not resolve a dilemma. The working through of a simple or complex problem can help us see something afresh and give us insights into our own or other people's difficulties. William Blake's poem *A Poison Tree* is a good example.

A Poison Tree

I was angry with my friend:
I told my wrath, my wrath did end.
I was angry with my foe:
I told it not, my wrath did grow.

And I water'd it in fears,
Night & morning with my tears;
And I sunned it with smiles,
And with soft deceitful wiles.

And it grew both day and night,
Till it bore an apple bright;
And my foe beheld it shine,
And he knew that it was mine,

And into my garden stole
When the night had veil'd the pole:
In the morning glad I see

My foe outstretch'd beneath the tree.
(William Blake)

The poem illustrates beautifully the consequences of unexpressed hostility – the growing anger, the deceitfulness and the fearfulness. What is fascinating about the poem is that it predates Freud by about a hundred years in articulating the harmful effects of repression. The most important part of Freud's work was his assertion that unacknowledged, censored feelings and fantasies continue to exercise a huge influence on our behaviour and are the major cause of neuroses.

Language of poetry

Poetry, more than any other literary form, is about sounds, images and rhythm. People would not read it if it *only* conveyed a thought or a feeling. Through the rhythm, sounds and imagery our imaginations are set alive and stretched. Dylan Thomas (1951), when responding to a query about what had influenced him to become a poet, wrote:

> I wanted to write poetry in the beginning because I had fallen in love with words. The words, 'Ride a cock-horse to Banbury Cross' were as haunting to me, who did not know what a cock-horse was, nor cared a damn where Banbury Cross might be, as, much later, were such lines as John Donne's 'Go and catch a falling star, Get with child a mandrake root' which also I could not understand when I first read them.[3]

Thomas captures something here about the essence of poetry: how much of it taps into our pre-conscious. It can connect with us in fragments, it can draw us in at the level of rhythm, or by a striking image. Nor is it frivolous to wonder why Thomas mentions that particular nursery rhyme; it has much that a fine poem should have:

> Ride a cock horse to Banbury Cross
> To see a fine lady ride on a white horse
> With rings on her fingers and bells on her toes
> She shall have music wherever she goes.

The rhythm enacts the soothing motion of a horse or a rocking horse, 'With rings on her fingers and bells on her toes' evokes sounds and sights, and 'She shall have music wherever she goes' gives a wonderful idea of infinite possibilities!

Rhythm can make our pulses go faster or slower, and we now know much more about the way physical processes can affect mental processes. A lot of modern poetry, in particular, uses rhythm to convey not just smoothness or rocking, but a sense of fragmentation, or a sense of dislocation or strangeness. In this way it resonates with the poet's thoughts and conveys the mood of the poem.

Writing poetry

The first section of this book is about links between therapeutic ideas and *established* poets, that is, those who have been published. However, one of the therapeutic aspects of reading and hearing poetry is how often it leads to people wanting to express themselves through writing poetry, especially when they are experiencing emotional distress. This does not seem to be the case for other literary forms. Reading novels does not usually lead to an outpouring of would-be novelists, or theatre-going to people wanting to become playwrights. Undoubtedly this has something to do with the fact that poetry is immediately accessible: a poem can express powerful feelings and thoughts in a direct, short format. It then seems to encourage something in other people to feel that they, too, could find a cathartic release in expressing themselves through poetry. Many people going through bereavement or faced with cancer or in mental health settings have been enormously helped by this means and the second section of the book explores this.

Poetry and therapy: similarities

To the extent that all art seeks to communicate, it would be true to say that therapy has something in common with all literary forms. The novel, with its development of character and plot and its narrative form, resembles the part of therapy that 'tells the story' and begs the question of 'what will happen next'. Some people's lives seem to resemble a novel, with eccentric or warring parents, jealous siblings, figures who rescue or abandon, and incredible coincidences. Drama is a wonderful medium for exploring communication between individuals. It shows intimate communication, miscommunication, dysfunctional communication and the ebb and flow of tension between characters. But, for me, poetry is the literary form that is most *like* therapy.

A poem can start with an image like a rock, a tulip, a railway station or a shoe box, and from that image layers of meaning emerge. Similarly, a client may start, 'I don't know why I feel so down today. I just dropped my son off at school: nothing was different, just he didn't turn back and wave as he usually does'. From that tiny detail may come a sensation of not being needed as a parent in the same way, linked to a powerful memory of not being wanted, to an overwhelming feeling of isolation. The therapeutic relationship gives space and the right climate for deeper levels of meaning to be explored. In the example I have given it starts to make sense to the client why such a seemingly trivial event can lead to a deep sense of isolation.

Revealing deeper layers of feeling can lead to a cathartic experience where the person can feel and then express a deep sense of anger, loss or shame; feelings that they usually defend themselves from experiencing, let alone expressing. Cathartic means cleansing, and the individual in therapy may feel that by expressing these feelings in a safe setting they have 'cleansed' or 'cleared out' these powerful feelings. They no longer have the power to go on affecting their lives in the same way. Poets often write for the same reason: in expressing powerful feelings, they can then let go of them. Graham Greene described writing as a form of therapy, saying, 'I wonder how all those who do not write, compose or paint can manage to escape the madness, melancholia, the panic fear which is inherent in the human situation'.

Not only do literature and therapy seek to communicate, they both explicitly see words as a means of transformation. In *Macbeth* Malcolm urges Macduff to express his grief:

> Give sorrow words: the grief that does not speak,
> Whispers the o'er-fraught heart, and bids it break.
> (*Macbeth*, 1606, Act IV, Scene 3)

And in a similar tone, in *Twelfth Night* Viola, describing a love suppressed, says:

> She never told her love,
> But let concealment, like a worm i' the bud,
> Feed on her damask cheek
> (*Twelfth Night*, 1601, Act II, Scene 4)

It is easy to see why Freud had such a high regard for Shakespeare. Like Blake, he had an instinctive feeling for psychological truths.

Authenticity

Implicit in this notion of stripping away layers is the idea that people *want* to be their 'authentic selves'. Carl Rogers talks of therapy as enabling people to move from an incongruent to a congruent way of being; psychodynamic therapy aims to help clients form a strong enough ego so that they no longer need to use defences in such a dysfunctional way; Winnicott coined the expression the 'true and the false self'. Cognitive behavioural therapy encourages people to replace unrealistic beliefs with more realistic beliefs. The heart of transpersonal therapy is to help people connect with their real or spiritual centre.

Many poets, particularly modern poets, would lay claim to the same goal, that of finding a true and authentic voice. Seamus Heaney (2002)[4] describes poetry as 'revelation of the self to the self'.

Linked to the idea of being authentic is that of being self-aware: it is hard to be authentic if you don't know how you really feel. Many things can happen to estrange people from their 'true selves'. They may have internalised values, particularly those of parents, which are not their own values: feelings like joy or anger may have been censored and smothered at an early age.

All therapies place a high value on self-awareness but Gestalt therapy uses the concept in a way that is particularly akin to ideas of creativity. *Gestalt*, a German word, roughly translates as 'pattern' or 'meaningful whole'. Gestalt therapy, developed by Fritz and Laura Perls, visualises our physical, emotional and cognitive lives as continually producing needs that come into our awareness. This could be a very simple need, such as an awareness of being thirsty. The individual becomes aware that his throat is dry, he then decides to do something to meet that need, so he gets a drink of water. He drinks the water and the need is met. It then fades into the background, the *gestalt* is complete, but soon another need will arise.

More complicated needs, like the need for affection or the need to express anger, may not move so easily from the sensation of awareness to the satisfying of the need. The individual may censor the awareness at an early stage or may constantly sabotage his own attempts to move from awareness to action. The *gestalt* is therefore incomplete. Much of Gestalt therapy is concerned with working with a client to help him become more aware of what he is suppressing.

This cycle of awareness has obvious parallels with the creative process that impels the writer from the moment of awareness to that of completion. It accords with Robert Frost's (1923) remark:

> A poem begins with a lump in the throat; a home-sickness or a love-sickness. It is a reaching-out toward expression; an effort to find fulfilment. A complete poem is one where an emotion has found its thought and the thought has found the words.[5]

Robert Frost's remark expresses eloquently the culmination of feeling and thought into a creative work, which then brings a sense of completion. For me, it also brings to mind a similar feeling in individual or group therapy when something authentic and important is expressed. A poet completes the cycle of awareness by the writing of the poem. A client goes through a similar process when there is a real meeting of heart, mind and self-discovery through the therapeutic relationship.

Ted Hughes' poem *The Thought Fox* is an almost perfect demonstration of a completed *gestalt*. It also brings together physical senses, thoughts and feelings in a powerful way, an important feature of Gestalt therapy:

The Thought Fox

I imagine this midnight moment's forest:
Something else is alive
Beside the clock's loneliness
And this blank page where my fingers move.

Through the window I see no star:

Something more near
Though deeper within darkness
Is entering the loneliness:

Cold, delicately as the dark snow
A fox's nose touches twig, leaf;
Two eyes serve a movement, that now
And again now, and now, and now

Sets neat prints into the snow
Between trees, and warily a lame
Shadow lags by stump and in hollow
Of a body that is bold to come

Across clearings, an eye,
A widening, deepening greenness,
Brilliantly, concentratedly,
Coming about its own business

Till, with a sudden sharp hot stink of fox,
It enters the dark hole of the head.
The window is starless still; the clock ticks,
The page is printed.[6]
(Ted Hughes)

Dreams and unconscious processes

Dreams have often featured in literary works – as wish fulfilment, warning, prophecy or magic. Whatever cultural belief they reflect, they frequently come across as deeply imaginative with rich imagery. In the Old Testament of The Bible the Pharaoh dreams of seeing seven sleek, fat cows, followed by seven thin cows. Joseph interprets this to mean that there will be seven good harvests followed by seven years of harvest failures.

Freud, in an age of scientific enquiry, brought dreams back into the arena of something deeply serious and worthy of attention. Twentieth-century writers have usually reflected his view that, in some way, the dream represents a part of the individual's psyche, unconscious wishes or desires.

Freud and Jung differed considerably in the way they regarded dreams. Freud thought the dream contained the repressed, forbidden sexual or aggressive drive that the conscious mind could not permit. It was in interpreting what lay behind the 'latent' content that revealed to the patient a source of psychological tension and anxiety. Jung came to understand dreams as the psyche's drive towards health and thought that the conscious, waking self could almost be instructed, guided or enriched by experiencing and then accepting the dream. A poem that illustrates these ideas is Thom Gunn's *The Reassurance*:

The Reassurance

About ten days or so
After we saw you dead
You came back in a dream.
I'm all right now you said.

And it *was* you, although
You were fleshed out again:
You hugged us all round then,
And gave your welcoming beam.

How like you to be kind,
Seeking to reassure.
And, yes, how like my mind
To make itself secure.[7]
(Thom Gunn)

This simple but poignant poem reflects the Jungian idea of healing taking place both in the dream itself and in the telling of the dream.

It is not only dreams that have influenced twentieth-century writers. Anthony Storr (1989) says:

> During the twentieth century, psychoanalysis had a major effect upon both art and literature. Freud's concept of the unconscious, his use of free association, and his rediscovery of the importance of dreams encouraged painters, sculptors, and writers to experiment with the fortuitous and the irrational, to pay serious attention to their inner worlds of dream and day-dream, and to find significance in thoughts and images that they would previously have dismissed as absurd or illogical.[8]

James Joyce and Virginia Wolf employed the 'stream of consciousness' approach to writing, one thought or image giving rise to another, sometimes in seemingly illogical ways. It is hard to think of T S Eliot's 'The Wasteland' being written without the knowledge that fragmented thoughts and images – which only make sense if we allow that unconscious processes are at play – do add up to a whole.

Therapists' view of creativity

Anthony Storr's chapter entitled 'Art and Literature' in his introductory book on Freud[8] gives a very perceptive account of what he calls Freud's 'curiously ambivalent attitude to art and artists'. On the one hand, Freud had a deep love of and knowledge of literature. He acknowledged the very special gifts of artists and writers, yet 'Freud believed that the sublimation of unsatisfied libido was responsible for producing all art and literature'.

In his paper *Creative Writers and Day Dreaming* (Freud, 1908) Freud writes:

The creative writer does the same as the child at play. He creates a world of phantasy which he takes very seriously – that is which he invests with large amounts of emotion – while separating it sharply from reality.[9]

The phantasy, in Freud's view, would always be a sign of some immaturity or unhappiness, for he continues:

We may lay it down that a happy person never phantasies, only an unsatisfied one. The motive forces of phantasies are unsatisfied wishes.[9]

Storr[8] comments that if Freud had lived longer he might have been influenced by biologists who saw play, the precursor to fantasy, as a necessary and helpful developmental step. Much scientific breakthrough is made simply because scientists allow their minds to play and fantasise. Certainly, those therapists who followed in Freud's footsteps and modified his theories have a much more positive attitude towards the healthy aspect of the creative arts. Melanie Klein, in particular, saw creativity as having a reparative function in the guilt the infant feels in its fantasised attack on the mother. If some of creative writing is concerned with an individual working out his own neurotic conflicts, that would be seen as a positive way of resolving difficulties.

Jung was always interested in the issue of creativity and encouraged his patients to paint and then talk about their work. In 1922 he gave a lecture to the Society for German Language and Literature entitled 'On the Relation of Analytical Psychology to Poetry'. He agrees with Freud in that he sees much of creative work arising from the unconscious but says:

The special significance of a true work of art resides in the fact that it has escaped from the limitations of the personal and has soared beyond the personal concerns of its creator.[10]

Carl Rogers, Abraham Maslow and the Gestalt therapists who form part of the Humanist School put a high value on creativity in the broadest definition of the word. They believed strongly that creativity is an inbuilt part of being human: therapy could often act to unblock the creative energy that is in each one of us. Rogers (1954) asks why it should matter whether people want to be conformist, rather than creative and answers his own question:

In a time when knowledge, constructive and destructive, is advancing by the most incredible leaps and bounds into a fantastic atomic age, genuinely creative adaptation seems to represent the only possibility that man can keep abreast of the kaleidoscopic change in his world. Unless individuals, groups and nations can imagine, construct and creatively revise new ways of relating to these complex changes, the lights will go out.[11]

Poets' views on therapy

It would be impossible to come to any collective view on how poets would view therapy: their views would be as diverse as the general population. We have seen the opinions of some poets as to why they write poetry – because they fell in love with words, as a cathartic experience, as a way of working out sad, mad or difficult feelings, or simply as a response to everything they experience in the world around them. Robert Frost's remark of a poem beginning as a lump in the throat captures that feeling of something arising in the writer which he or she then struggles to express and communicate, first to him or herself, then to other people.

Poets have had a reputation for being gloomy, intense, introverted, alcoholic, or wise and enlightened. It probably is not very helpful to categorise them. Some poets write in a highly autobiographical way; others attempt to communicate what they see as universal themes and keep their own personality removed. Neil Astley (2002), in his introduction to his poetry anthology *Staying Alive*, writes:

> Poets no longer live in ivory towers. Today's poets come from all kinds of backgrounds and cultures, women as well as men; they are much more tuned in to how people think about the world and feel about themselves than the poets of 50 years ago. What the best poets write is relevant to people's lives and to their experience of the world, on an everyday as well as on a more spiritual level.[12]

In other words, poets often have a wider experience of life, have done other jobs, and have not always defined themselves as 'a poet'. However, there may well be a feeling among some creative people that, by engaging in therapy, they would somehow 'dilute' their art. The psychological pain is part of their art and to 'treat' the pain would in some way diminish the art. I see this as a false view as I believe that most therapists see part of their role as supporting and encouraging the creative part of their clients, not explaining it away.

There is often a myth about therapy, that it 'cures' people, as a physical disease might be cured. Most therapists have a more realistic view that therapy is only a partial cure, or the beginning of a process to a happier, more fulfilled life. Therapy can help unblock channels of communication, it can open up the inner world so that it becomes more attuned to the outer world, it can encourage someone to have more belief in himself, but it does not fundamentally alter the individual. Nor is it something done 'to' an individual without his co-operation, but is a collaborative exploration.

Again, I can only marvel at Shakespeare's modernity. What doctor, nurse or therapist has not heard a desperate patient or relative say, like Macbeth, when viewing his wife's emotional disintegration:

> Canst thou not minister to a mind diseased?
> Pluck from the memory a rooted sorrow,
> Raze out the written troubles of the brain,
> And, with some sweet oblivious antidote,
> Cleanse the stuffed bosom of that perilous stuff
> Which weighs upon the heart?
> (*Macbeth*, Act V, Scene 3)

In other words, 'Isn't there something you can **do** for her?'. The doctor's reply, 'Therein the Patient/Must minister to himself', echoes the therapist's approach, probably more tactfully expressed, that the patient or client is going to have to do at least half of the work. There is no magical transformation.

Conclusion

I have looked at some of the similarities between writing and hearing poetry and what goes on in therapy and counselling. I have also suggested some of the reasons why people find poetry uplifting, instructive and therapeutic. In the next chapters I shall explore themes that are common to both poetry and therapy.

References

1 Alvarez A (2003) Quoted in foreword to H Canham and C Satyamurti (eds) *Acquainted with the Night: psychoanalysis and the poetic imagination*. Karnac, London.
2 Drew E (1959) *Poetry: a modern guide to its understanding and enjoyment*. WW Norland & Co.
3 Thomas D (1951) Quoted in C Fitzgibbon (1965) *The Life of Dylan Thomas*. Dent, London.
4 Heaney S (2002) *Finders Keepers*. Faber & Faber Ltd, London.
5 Frost R, in H Holt (ed.) (1923) *Robert Frost: the man and his work*. Henry Holt, New York.
6 Hughes T (1957) *The Thought Fox*. From *The Hawk in the Rain*. Faber & Faber Ltd, London.
7 Gunn T *The Reassurance*. From *The Man With Night Sweats*. Faber & Faber Ltd, London.
8 Storr A (1989) *Freud, A Very Brief Introduction*. Oxford University Press, Oxford.
9 Freud S (1908) Creative writers and day dreaming. In: Strachey J (ed.) (1990) *The Penguin Freud Library, Volume 14: art and literature*. Penguin, Harmondsworth.
10 Jung C (1922) On the relation of analytical psychology to poetry. In: *Jung, The Spirit in Man, Art and Literature*. Routledge Classics, London.
11 Rogers C (1954) Towards a theory of creativity. In: Vernon PE (1970) *Creativity*. Penguin, Harmondsworth.
12 Astley N (2002) *Staying Alive*. Bloodaxe Books, Newcastle upon Tyne.

CHAPTER 2

Transitions in life: early stages

Life is lived forward but understood backward
(Kierkegaard)

It seems a cliché to say that our human lifespan is a series of stages: that we are born into this world, grow up, go to school, make friends, form or don't form adult partnerships, perhaps have children, work, retire, age and finally die. In Shakespeare's famous speech from *As You Like It* Jaques compresses all seven stages into 28 lines. This 'overview', combined with the metaphor of a stage play, gives the whole process a sense of brevity, distance and yet universality.

All the world's a stage,
And all the men and women merely players:
They have their exits and their entrances;
And one man in his time plays many parts,
His acts being seven ages. At first the infant,
Mewling and puking in the nurse's arms.
And then the whining schoolboy, with his satchel,
And shining morning face, creeping like a snail
Unwillingly to school. And then the lover,
Sighing like a furnace, with a woful ballad
Made to his mistress' eyebrow. Then a soldier,
Full of strange oaths, and bearded like the pard,
Jealous in honour, sudden and quick in quarrel,
Seeking the bubble reputation
Even in the cannon's mouth.
And then the justice,
In fair round belly with good capon lin'd,
With eyes severe, and beard of formal cut,
Full of wise saws and modern instances;
And so he plays his part. The sixth age shifts
Into the lean and slipper'd pantaloon,
With spectacles on nose and pouch on side,
His youthful hose well sav'd, a world too wide

For his shrunk shank; and his big manly voice,
Turning again toward childish treble, pipes
And whistles in his sound. Last scene of all,
That ends this strange eventful history,
Is second childishness and mere oblivion,
Sans teeth, sans eyes, sans taste, sans everything.
(*As You Like It*, 1599, Act II, Scene 7)

The next two chapters examine some of these life stages. When we are immersed in life these stages seldom seem clear or objective. Because it is such a vast subject I have chosen to focus on just three areas: in this chapter, adolescence, and in the next chapter, issues concerned with becoming a parent and middle age. It is often the changes brought about by moving into the next life stage that bring about problems, tensions and anxieties. Change in itself can be both challenging and stimulating, something to be anticipated: but it can also bring feelings of strangeness, insecurity or disappointment. Change, however desirable, always involves giving up something. Thinking about what is involved in some of these life stages may make it easier to see why they can be times of excitement and fulfilment, stress and self-doubt or a mixture of all these emotions.

Individuals often seek help from a therapist or counsellor when they feel something has gone wrong with the way they are coping or not coping with this new phase of their life. The new phase an individual enters often reactivates earlier problems he or she may have had. An example would be the birth of a child when the parent may re-experience feelings of possessiveness, or feel excluded in a triangular relationship.

Because writers tend to be sensitive to and interested in moments of upheaval and discovery rather than smooth waters, much is written in prose and poetry about transitions in life. Seldom does an autobiography bypass the pain, embarrassment and humour (usually retrospective) of adolescence. First love, becoming a parent, middle age and old age are topics that have been written about with tenderness, sensitivity and humour. Everyone's life is unique, yet everyone goes through this maturational process. When someone dies an untimely death, part of the grief is for the opportunity that person has lost to experience the full stretch of human existence.

Our bodies go through the process of birth, growth, maturation, ageing and death, but there are vast differences in how these life stages are regarded in different cultures. Each culture evolves its own values for male and female roles, determines who raises the children and how they are raised, ascribes high or low value to different stages of life – for instance old age. In the Eurocentric climate of the first half of the twentieth century, a time when many psychological theories were formed, cultural differences were largely ignored, and a great deal of reshaping of ideas has had to take place to accommodate very different child-rearing practices.

The idea of life stages

The psychologists who pay most attention to the concept of life stages – the emotional development that takes place and what helps or frustrates that process – are the psychodynamic thinkers: Freud, Jung, Klein, Adler and their followers. Freud conceptualised early infancy as a series of stages the baby, toddler and young child went through, naming them the oral, anal, oedipal and genital stage. Symbolically, they represent issues of dependency, control, rivalry and maturity. He believed that it was getting stuck or fixated in these stages that led to neurosis. The task of therapy was to help the patient resolve or become aware of conflicts arising from these developmental stages, but expressed in adult life.

Freud's groundbreaking work, which all psychodynamic practitioners have followed, was to observe, describe and then work with the unresolved conflicts that he perceived were being carried through into adult life. The conflict, which had originated in childhood, would be subtly played out in adult life. So, for example, a small boy who had remained stuck in an oedipal situation – an intense romantic attachment to his mother with a desire to exclude and (in fantasy) kill off his father – might carry through into adult life a pattern of perceiving and behaving as if every situation in life was one of competition with the need to annihilate competitors.

A century before Freud was writing about developmental processes, Wordsworth had written 'the child is father of the man', suggesting that childhood experience forms or shapes the adult. A poem where I think this is suggested, if not stated, is Hugo Williams' *Dinner with My Mother*:

Dinner with My Mother

My mother is saying 'Now'.
'Now,' she says, taking down a saucepan,
putting it on the stove.
She doesn't say anything else for a while,

so that time passes slowly, on the simmer,
until it is 'Now' again
as she hammers out our steaks
for Steak Diane.

I have to be on hand at times like this
for table-laying,
drink replenishment
and general conversational encouragement,

but I am getting hungry
and there is nowhere to sit down.
'Now,' I say, making a point
of opening a bottle of wine.

My mother isn't listening.
She's miles away,
testing the sauce with a spoon,
narrowing her eyes through the steam.

'Now,' she says very slowly, meaning
which is it to be,
the rosemary or tarragon vinegar
for the salad dressing?

I hold my breath, lest anything
should go wrong at the last minute.
But now it is really 'Now',
our time to sit and eat.[1]
(Hugo Williams)

There is no mention in this poem of links with childhood but it would not be fanciful to see a replaying of childhood preoccupations, such as 'When am I going to be fed?', 'Will my needs be taken care of?', 'Have I got my mother's attention?', and the poet's attempts – 'Now,' I say, making a point of opening a bottle of wine' – to exert some control over a situation in which he evidently feels quite powerless.

Erikson's view of life stages

Freud's primary focus of interest was in very early stages of a child's development, principally before the age of five. Erikson, an analyst in the Freudian school, built on Freud's ideas but developed them further, postulating that, throughout our lifetime, there are certain 'tasks' and challenges that a particular life stage throws up. Like Freud, he believed that satisfactory early childhood experiences were the building blocks of emotional health and that when people experienced problems it was usually because something from an earlier life stage had not been satisfactorily negotiated. Though some of his ideas of the roles in life expressed in his book *Childhood and Society*[2] now seem outdated, I think his concept of the tasks and preoccupations of each stage are still useful and valid.

Erikson's eight stages of development do not really match Shakespeare's as, being a post- Freudian thinker, he attributes much more importance to the stages of childhood. There is no exact measure of these stages, but this is what he postulates are the tasks of each stage:

Basic trust versus mistrust (first year of life).
Autonomy versus shame and doubt (two to three years).
Initiative versus guilt (four to five years).
Industry versus inferiority (five to 11 years).
Identity versus role confusion (adolescence).
Intimacy versus isolation (young adulthood).

Generativity versus stagnation (middle age).
Ego integrity versus despair (old age).

Thus, he sees the first 'task' or preoccupation of a baby is to come to terms with whether the world is basically a trustworthy place or not. This first foundation stone is shaped by whether, by and large, the baby's needs are met with love and consistency, he or she is fed regularly, feels the secure warmth and comfort of the mother or other caregiver and is not subjected to prolonged or frequent frustration. In addition, the baby needs to be sure that his or her caregiver is available and does not disappear. As the baby grows into a toddler he learns that he can say yes or no, co-operate or have a tantrum, comply or rebel. Issues of control and self-control become paramount. If parents can provide reasonably secure boundaries, allow some flexibility and yet safety and firmness, the child can start to develop a sense of himself (autonomy) without feeling shame or self-doubt.

This is not a book about child development but I quote these early stages to give an insight into the way that psychodynamic therapists view human development. However, I have chosen to focus on just one of Erikson's pre-adult life stages, that of adolescence, partly because so much literature links into that period of life.

Adolescence

This phase at the end of childhood, the beginning of sexual maturation, the transition between childhood and adulthood, has only comparatively recently been accorded a recognised name and timescale. It is interesting to see in Shakespeare's account the individual goes straight from the schoolboy with his satchel 'creeping like a snail unwillingly to school' to 'a lover with a woful ballad'. Western society, in recent years, recognises this prolonged period of time when the individual is neither a child nor an adult, which can last up to seven or eight years. During this time the young person gradually explores new roles and responsibilities, sexuality, skills, extends sporting and academic prowess, experiences friendships and romances, all within some framework of family and education. The choices and freedoms may seem enticing but it is hardly surprising they also act as a pressure on the young person.

In many other societies and in our pre-industrial society adolescence hardly existed. The transition from child to adult was rapid and prescribed. The following poem, by a contemporary East African poet, reflects a very definite set of values and expectations on a young person:

Come, My Mother's Son

Come, my mother's son
You're no longer a baby
Stop following the women

To the firesides
Stop peeping in the cooking pot
Stop pinching the girls
You're no longer a baby
You are a man

Come, my mother's son
Show your bravery
And step fully into manhood
The test is not hard
Not with determination

Let not the women chirp
And giggle in mockery
And call you names
Come, my mother's son
Show and prove your bravery
And rightfully claim your stand
Among the young warriors

My mother's son,
Shine your prowess
As a great warrior, a dancer
A great player, a sprinter
And get yourself admirers
Get a bride of your choice
Come, my mother's son
Let's see your test

Come, my mother's son
Heed to prove your manhood
Cultivate the trees of your forefathers
For a continual bloom and fruit bearing
Carry on your father's name into the future
Come, my mother's son
Cower not, stand as a man
And let us see you are a man.[3]
(Lillian Ingonga)

There may be adolescents and parents who wish that *our* society was as clear in its expectations of a young person as the author of this poem, and would respond positively to the defined future earmarked for this young man. Many adolescents today face a good deal of uncertainty about the direction in which they are travelling educationally, morally and in family relationships.

Erikson's view of adolescence: identity versus role confusion

Erikson describes the adolescent phase as one where the young person is seeking to affirm or discover his or her identity and where, implicitly, there is a great deal of confusion about his or her role. Do I want to be like or different from my parents? Do I want to forge a close, intimate relationship with someone or remain part of a larger group? What clothes, make-up and style shall I pursue? What will make me acceptable to my peers and whose rules and mores do I now live by? These are almost impossible questions to answer without a lot of questioning, rebellion, self-doubt, bravado and experimentation, and when adolescence is portrayed in novels, films, poetry and biography, it is usually poignant, sometimes humorous. Some of the best novels of the 1940s and 1950s, such as *Catcher in the Rye* by J D Salinger and *The Member of the Wedding* by Carson McCullers (1946), have an adolescent as their main character. *The Member of the Wedding* begins:

> It happened that green and crazy summer when Frankie was twelve years old. This was the summer when for a long time she had not been a member. She belonged to no club and was a member of nothing in the world. Frankie had become an unjoined person who hung around in doorways and she was afraid. This summer she was grown so tall that she was almost a big freak, and her shoulders were narrow, her legs too long.[4]

This is a story of a particularly isolated young girl, whose mother died some years previously, but I believe it captures the discomfort and anxiety of some adolescents. Another American writer, Gwendolyn Brooks, describes the importance of the clan or group and the point of 'hanging out', beloved by teenagers and a source of annoyance for a lot of adults:

We Real Cool

The Pool Players
Seven at the Golden Shovel

We real cool.
We Left school. We

Lurk late.
We Strike straight. We
Sing sin. We
Thin gin. We

Jazz June. We
Die soon.[5]
(Gwendolyn Brooks)

This poem resonates the energy, rhythm, bravado and self-dramatising aspects of adolescence. The school drop-outs affirm their identity in a defiant but seemingly self-confident way. In an interview Brooks describes seeing these youngsters in a poolroom when they should have been in school and feeling that their identity was a little less sure than the one they were projecting. This is reflected in the last lines:

> We
> Die soon.

If, as Erikson says, adolescents are wrestling with finding a new identity, the group is often the only setting in which they can feel secure. At the same time the young person knows this can be a fragile security since groups can form and also break up. To be effective the group may feel compelled to adopt different values and mores from the adults. As Erikson says:

> In their search for a new sense of continuity and sameness, adolescents have to re-fight many of the battles of earlier years, even though to do so they must artificially appoint perfectly well-meaning people to play the roles of adversaries.[2]

The search for a new identity, often done deliberately provocatively, sometimes executed with false bravado, is beautifully described in the following poem:

For Heidi with Blue Hair

When you dyed your hair blue
(or, at least, ultramarine
for the clipped sides, with a crest
of jet-black spikes on top)
you were sent home from school

because, as the headmistress put it,
although dyed hair was not
specifically forbidden, yours
was, apart from anything else,
not done in the school colours.

Tears in the kitchen, telephone-calls
to school from your freedom-loving father:
'She's not a punk in her behaviour;
it's just a style.' (You wiped your eyes,
also not in a school colour.)

'She discussed it with me first –

we checked the rules.' 'And anyway, Dad,
it cost twenty-five dollars.
Tell them it won't wash out –
not even if I wanted to try.'

It would have been unfair to mention
your mother's death, but that
shimmered behind the arguments.
The school had nothing else against you;
the teachers twittered and gave in.

Next day your black friend had hers done
in grey, white and flaxen yellow –
the school colours precisely:
an act of solidarity, a witty
tease. The battle was already won.[6]
(Fleur Adcock)

This poem conjures up the battlefield that exists in adolescence, though in this case the parent is the ally and the school the enemy. However, even they are shown to be able to adapt, and the death of the mother, just alluded to, hints at the very real additional burdens that face some young people going through what is already a turbulent time. The poem also captures the volatile nature of adolescence: the young girl is striking out on her individual path, but desperately needs her father when it all goes wrong!

Rebellion against authority, yet extreme conformity within the chosen group, characterises adolescent behaviour. This is why young people often appear to be quite cruel to those outside the group who show any difference. Young people who have no group to belong to experience real misery in adolescence and, as they are at the same time trying to establish some independence from their parents, often feel isolated and adrift. Conversely, if an adolescent has a supportive group that offers him or her a strong sense of belonging he or she can weather painful experiences at home.

Specific difficulties in adolescence

Most adolescents will experience upheaval, anxiety about their appearance, conflict between different sets of standards and ambivalence about growing up. Winnicott's (1965) famous remark was that 'the only real cure for adolescence is the passage of time'.[7] However, there are two scenarios that make these years a particularly difficult and stressful time. The first is when difficult life events are also going on in the young person's life. These include things such as sad and acrimonious separations between parents, death or serious illness of a parent, sibling or other close family member, being bullied at school and a feeling of having no friends. The two novels I mentioned, *Catcher in the Rye* and *The Member of the Wedding*, are both set after a family bereavement. In *Catcher in the Rye* Holden Caulfield's seemingly perfect and popular brother, Allie, has died of leukaemia and in *The Member of the Wedding* Frankie's mother is dead. In both novels there is a huge hole at the centre of the character's inner life, which makes them extremely painful books to read.

The other scenario is when those early life stages of dependence, autonomy, engagement with learning and a sense of independence and confidence have been shakily or unhappily passed through. Ellen Noonan (1984) says:

> It is essential for the counsellor to be able to distinguish between those who are having to find themselves for the first time and those who are merely having to reshape themselves, that is, between those who have never felt firmly grounded in their own experience and can't say 'I am' with any conviction, and those who know who they are despite confusion, anxiety and change.[8]

Young people from these two scenarios may come to the attention of psychologists or counsellors, often as a result of their behaviour: withdrawn, aggressive, self-harming, delinquent or showing signs of an eating disorder. Drug or alcohol abuse may be a symptom or a cause of other problems. However, many unhappy teenagers never come near any sort of professional services. Creative work in school – both their own endeavours and in being introduced to artistic work – can be the most sustaining aspect of their emotional life.

Nicholas Mazza (2003),[9] in his chapter on poetry therapy and adolescent suicide, cautions that, although poems which reflect the difficult and troubled mood of an adolescent are helpful, they should always have a positive message and suggest that a positive direction is possible. He quotes Leedy (1969),[10] who says that with depressed and potentially suicidal clients poems that offer no hope, increase guilt, or advocate the seeking of vengeance should not be used.

Conclusion

Some young people pass through the stage of adolescence relatively smoothly and seem to have a very mature vision of how life will be for them when they become fully adult. Most, though, experience upheaval that is challenging and at times bewildering. Some young people are extremely unhappy and depressed throughout this period. If adults want to reach out to help and support them, they have to find a means of communication that appeals to the young person. Music, song lyrics and accessible literature are often forms that are less threatening, especially at the beginning point of contact. Encouraging original writing in young people, both in looking within themselves and to the outside world, can make an enormous contribution in giving voice to the energy and confusion that are part of most adolescents' experience. Suggestions as to how to work with young people will be found in Part 2 of this book.

References

1 Williams H (1992) *Dinner with My Mother*. From *Collected Poems*. Faber & Faber Ltd, London.
2 Erikson E (1950) *Childhood and Society*. Vintage, London.
3 Ingonga L (1988) *Come, My Mother's Son*. From AD Amateshe *An Anthology of East African Poetry*. Longman Press, Harlow, Essex.
4 McCullers C (1946) *The Member of the Wedding*. Penguin Books, Harmondsworth.
5 Brooks G *We Real Cool*. From *Collected Poems*. Harper Collins Publishers.
6 Adcock F (2000) *For Heidi with Blue Hair*. From *Poems 1960–2000*. Bloodaxe Books, London.
7 Winnicott DW (1965) *The Family and Individual Development*. Tavistock Publications, London.
8 Noonan E (1984) *Counselling Young People*. Sage Publications, London.
9 Mazza N (2003) *Poetry Therapy*. Brunner-Routledge, Hove.
10 Leedy JJ (1969) Principles of poetry. In: Leedy JJ (ed.) *The Use of Poetry in the Treatment of Emotional Disorders*. Lippincott, Philadelphia, USA.

CHAPTER 3

Transitions in life: later stages

In this chapter, still using Erikson's framework, I shall look at two of the life stages in adulthood – becoming a parent and middle age. 'Things end, there is a time of fertile emptiness and then things begin anew', writes William Bridges (1980),[1] reinforcing the point in the last chapter that change involves giving up as well as gaining something.

The birth of a child

There are few experiences that bring change in such a dramatic way as the birth of a child. Adolescence, middle age, old age may creep up gradually, have several defining moments, but a baby is in the womb one day, and a living, kicking, demanding, hungry being the next. Becoming a parent is life changing. For the mother, the physical, biological, hormonal changes are immense; for both parents the emotional journey is huge and rapid.

Most parents experience feelings of joy, pride and protectiveness towards their baby, but some also feel moved by more universal feelings of awe and wonder, connecting them to deep issues of life, death and creativity. In Chapter 4 I suggest that these deep feelings can lead to a sense of altruism, or to a feeling that material values are unimportant. This takes many parents by surprise: the depth of their feelings can lead to a willingness to make sacrifices and a sense of commitment they had not previously experienced.

Although Erikson's phase of 'Intimacy versus Isolation', that of early adulthood, refers primarily to the forming of a stable partnership, he also describes it as a stage of life where the individual is:

> ready for intimacy, that is, the capacity to commit himself to concrete affiliations and partnerships and to develop the ethical strength to abide by such commitments, even though they may call for significant sacrifices and compromises.[2]

Most parents have thought about this commitment but the enormity of it forces itself onto them in the very helplessness and neediness of the baby. The response may be one of extreme love and protectiveness, fulfilment and optimism. There may also be feelings of panic, inadequacy or fear for the future, but it is rare that a parent feels neutral. Indeed, it is because of the knowledge, conscious or unconscious, that momentous feelings are called for, that a parent, particularly a mother, feels a great sense of emotional devastation or inadequacy if she feels cut off or dissociated from positive feelings about her baby.

Many poems have been written about those first weeks of parenthood. Milton, Coleridge and Yeats all wrote poems to their children, and contemporary poets such as Sylvia Plath and Sharon Olds express the intensity of their feelings at this time. This poem, by Sharon Olds, also speaks of the sense of fragility of a newborn baby, reinforcing the immense feeling of responsibility:

Her First Week

She was so small I would scan the crib a half-second
to find her, face-down in a corner, limp
as something gently flung down, or fallen
from some sky an inch above the mattress. I would
tuck her arm along her side
and slowly turn her over. She would tumble
over part by part, like a load
of damp laundry in the dryer, I'd slip
a hand in, under her neck,
slide the other under her back,
and evenly lift her up. Her little bottom
sat in my palm, her chest contained
the puckered, moire, sacs, and her neck –
I was afraid of her neck, once I almost
thought I heard it quietly snap,
I looked at her and she swivelled her slate
eyes and looked at me. It was in
my care, the creature of her spine, like the first
chordate, as if, history
of the vertebrate had been placed in my hands.
Every time I checked, she was still
with us – someday, there would be a human
race. I could not see it in her eyes,
but when I fed her, gathered her
like a loose bouquet to my side and offered
the breast, greyish-white, and struck with
miniscule scars like creeks in sunlight, I
felt she was serious, I believed she was willing to stay.[3]
(Sharon Olds)

Parental anxieties

The fearful, wondering and protective feelings described in this poem can be seen as the basis of bonding or attachment of a parent towards her or his baby. Perhaps this anxiety of whether your child is 'willing to stay' continues throughout parenthood and becomes transmuted into fear of illness, worries about harm from strangers or accidents on motor bikes. These first weeks and months as a parent of a new baby usually give rise to feelings of particular intensity. Winnicott (1965) talks about 'plunging into this extraordinary condition which is almost like an illness, though it is very much a sign of health'.[4]

But, as the baby and then child grows, the role of the parent requires not only nurturing, but encouragement to the child to engage in the outside world. Winnicott goes on to describe a damaging environment for both parent and child when the baby becomes 'her pathological preoccupation' so that neither can grow to become separate from each other. Bowlby's work in attachment theory talked of the need for the secure base for the child from which to explore its environment.

Tension between protectiveness, on the one hand, and independence, on the other, are not the only polarities parents face. Most parents have strong feelings of love, pride and joy in their baby mixed with feelings of resentment at the demands the baby and young child make. There are also worries about whether they are 'getting it right'. These ambivalent feelings are often very painful for parents who can feel bad or guilty when their feelings for their children are less than ideal, when they see bad traits in their children, or find their behaviour unmanageable. This can then become a vicious circle in that they criticise, punish or withdraw love, which tends to make the child's behaviour even worse. Therapeutic work can be so valuable in helping parents to express hostile, or mixed feelings about their children in a safe setting. This can often help them to get in touch with the more positive and resourceful aspects of themselves as a parent.

Being a parent involves being intimately involved in watching a little person grow, laugh, scream, develop language, understand and misunderstand words, learn it can comply or have a tantrum, discover many exciting things in its world and respond to its family, books, animals, food, all in a unique way. Change is happening all the time and this is exciting for parents, though there can also be a sense of loss, as each stage is abandoned for the next one. Many poems about parenthood seem to reflect this unique and precious journey. The poem is often similar to a photograph, freezing a particular moment in time:

Beattie is Three

At the top of the stairs
I ask for her hand. O.K.
She gives it to me.
How her fist fits my palm,

A bunch of consolation.
We take our time
Down the steep carpetway
As I wish silently
That the stairs were endless.[5]
(Adrian Mitchell)

The poem suggests to me that the poet wishes the stairs to be endless because of the perfection or completeness of the experience. It is a beautiful and simple poem, and illustrates the point I made earlier about attachment being a two-way process. The child needs and depends on its parents, but the parent is somehow made to feel complete by the child. Many novels have as their theme the overprotective parent, for example *Sons and Lovers* by D H Lawrence, but these are scenarios where the parent lives their life through their children or where they are blind to their child's need for separateness. In the real life experience of raising children it is the parent's empathy for their child that recognises this need for separation. But it is hardly surprising that, having experienced this intense emotional connection with a child, the bonds remain strong throughout life. Part of the 'ethical commitment' Erikson described is an understanding that a parent's role is also to help his or her child to become independent.

A poem by C Day Lewis captures that sense of almost physical pain that a parent can feel, at any stage of his child's life, when he realises the child has taken another step towards being a separate individual:

Walking Away – for Sean

It is eighteen years ago, almost to the day –
A sunny day with the leaves just turning,
The touch-lines new-ruled – since I watched you play
Your first game of football, then, like a satellite
Wrenched from its orbit, go drifting away

Behind a scatter of boys, I can see
You walking away from me towards the school
With the pathos of a half-fledged thing set free
Into a wilderness, the gait of one
Who finds no path where the path should be.

That hesitant figure, eddying away
Like a winged seed loosened from its parent stem
Has something I never quite grasp to convey
About nature's give-and-take – the small, the scorching
Ordeals which fire one's irresolute clay.

I have had worse partings, but none that so

Gnaws at my mind still. Perhaps it is roughly
Saying what God alone could perfectly show –
How selfhood begins with a walking away,
And love is proved in the letting go.[6]
(C Day Lewis)

The strength of this poem lies, I think, in the recognition that the striving for independence is one that both parent and young person make. The child needs to walk away, the parent proves his love by 'letting go'. The use of natural images such as the fledgling, the winged seed also imply 'it is in the nature of things' that this process happens. The feelings around this process can become very confused. A young person may be very fearful of freedom and project onto the parents that they are being unreasonably controlling. Parents, fearful of their child's independence, may exaggerate the dangers of the outside world, and thus convey mixed messages.

Middle age

John Betjeman, in his later years, was asked if there was anything he regretted in his life. With little hesitation and in his well-bred English voice he replied, 'Not enough sex'. I have often wondered whether the interviewer's jaw dropped or whether he carried on as smoothly as if Sir John had said, 'Yes, I always wish I had developed a more innovative approach to the tetrameter'.

Middle age is a time when people tend to evaluate their lives. People in this life stage know that more of their life is in the past tense than the future and there are some things they wanted from life that, realistically, they are unlikely to get. Like John Betjeman, with his sense that he didn't have enough sex, people may feel they haven't had enough love, enough money, haven't taken enough risks, haven't received the education they would have liked, have made poor decisions – the list is endless. People who have lived their lives like Dickens' Mr Micawber, in the belief that 'something will turn up', are faced with the strong possibility that maybe it won't.

These are of course perceptions, and perceptions are not facts but are subjective views. Counselling with people in middle age often focuses on what is a real loss and is irretrievable and what could, with a different perspective, be a possibility for a positive change. Middle age is also a time when evaluation of your life can involve great happiness and a sense of achievement. Certain worries and concerns can be relinquished. Elaine Feinstein's poem reflects some of this feeling:

Getting Older

The first surprise: I like it
Whatever happens now, some things
That used to terrify have not:

I didn't die young, for instance. Or lose
My only love. My three children
Never had to run away from anyone.

Don't tell me gratitude is complacent.
We all approach the edge of the same blackness
Which for me is silent.

Knowing as much sharpens
My delight in January freesia,
Hot coffee, winter sunlight, So we say

As we lie close on some gentle occasion:
Every day won from such
Darkness is a celebration.[7]
(Elaine Feinstein)

The overriding quality of this poem seems to me that of acceptance, not in a passive but in an active form, and a huge joy of living in the present. The wintry imagery suggests the dying down of life and the poem also raises a large issue of middle age, that of coming to terms with our mortality and the death of those we love. She talks of approaching 'the edge of the same blackness, which for me is silent'. She is using the realisation of her mortality, including the fact that she has no belief in an afterlife, as a fact that increases her appreciation of the everyday things of life.

Adjustment in middle age

Erikson alluded to this phase of life as 'Generativity versus Stagnation' and Jung (1931)[8] saw the lifespan as dividing into two: that leading up to middle age and the second half from middle age onwards. He describes this second phase as potentially a crisis phase if the individual cannot adapt to its demands. He felt that the individual needed to make a shift from preoccupation with the outer world to one that included a concern for meaning and spiritual values.

Adjustment to the idea that at least half of one's life is behind us is a mental process. Another process that goes on in middle age is that of adjusting to a changed body: changes in skin, hair and body tone and, for women, that one is no longer fertile. Given the massive attention to perfect, youthful bodies in the media, the emphasis on fitness and slimness, it would be surprising if many middle-aged people could view these changes without regret. Selima Hill's poem *Being Fifty* is an anarchic and imaginative poem that uses the image of a fridge to represent her body – large, cold and alien. She then fantasises about escaping across the ocean, though by now she has turned into a sofa:

Being Fifty

Being fifty makes me feel large,
large and cold like someone else's fridge.
I harbour scarlet fish
and fat gold eggs
that men in suits
with hands like vets'
remove.
I never speak.
Sometimes I might hum.
Or very rarely
raise a strangled gurgle
as if I'm trying one last time to lurch forward,
to get my fluff-clogged ankles
free from the lino,
hone myself, develop a fluked tail,
acquire a taste for frogbit,
and push off –
paddle off across the world's wide oceans
like a flat-footed sofa that's suddenly learnt how to swim,
piled high with jellies, cheeses, cushions,
fishes, poodles, babies, balding men,
swimming-pools, airing cupboards, hospitals,
and tiny pills, like polystyrene granules,
people advise one, or not,
to start taking.[9]
(Selima Hill)

This poem is full of images, apart from the obvious metaphors of the fridge and the sofa, some of them quite disturbing. It does, for me, capture a feeling of this age being a last opportunity to escape from a passive role into a richer landscape. These images are ones that could be very fruitful to work with in a therapy session and as a stimulus in a creative writing class. Does it represent a feeling of being trapped, of not being heard (the fridge is silent), manipulated by men, a determination to experience life before it is too late? The realisation that we are not immortal can be a helpful prod to make us get on and achieve things we have always wanted to. A counsellor can play an invaluable part in enabling a client to look at their dreams and aspirations and explore, in a supportive climate, which ones they feel they could still achieve and which ones may need to be relinquished. People who reach middle age at the beginning of the twenty-first century are fortunate that there are many role models around who defy the stereotypes of middle and old age as being a time to hang up your boots.

I said that middle age is a time of evaluation of your life and that includes whether you feel you have been fortunate or been dealt a poor hand of cards. There are undoubtedly great variations of fortune, in physical and mental health, disability, financial situation, how children have developed, whether there are grandchildren and if that is proving a satisfying role. Marriages are often re-evaluated once children have grown up.

Jenny Joseph's poem *Warning* is usually seen as a poem about old age because it starts with the words: 'When I am an old woman ...', but I see it as a poem about middle age. The woman speaking in the poem is both looking back on how she behaved in her youth and day-dreaming about the future, in the way we do when we're immersed in a settled present:

Warning

When I am an old woman I shall wear purple
With a red hat which doesn't go, and doesn't suit me,
And I shall spend my pension on brandy and summer gloves
And satin sandals, and say we've no money for butter.
I shall sit down on the pavement when I'm tired
And gobble up samples in shops and press alarm bells
And run my stick along the public railings
And make up for the sobriety of my youth.
I shall go out in my slippers in the rain
And pick the flowers in other people's gardens
And learn to spit.

You can wear terrible shirts and grow more fat
And eat three pounds of sausages at a go
Or only bread and pickle for a week
And hoard pens and pencils and beermats and things in boxes.

But now we must have clothes that keep us dry
And pay our rent and not swear in the street
And set a good example for the children.
We must have friends to dinner and read the papers.

But maybe I ought to practise a little now?
So people who know me are not too shocked and surprised
When suddenly I am old, and start to wear purple.[10]
(Jenny Joseph)

The poem is a wonderful antidote to the 'stagnation' that Erikson talks about. I think it reflects a value inherent in counselling and therapy, that change is always a creative possibility. As Rogers would say, the counsellor is there to provide the right conditions, the right soil for an individual to experience his or her fullest and most authentic self. Or, as George Eliot said, 'It is never too late to be what you might have been'. Self-expression through writing also seems to be a particularly powerful medium for this age group.

Conclusion

It is always valuable to know why someone has decided to approach a counsellor at a particular moment of his or her life. Even if the reason may appear to be as a response to external life events, such as divorce or bereavement, issues often arise connected with that particular life stage. The life journey for each of us is unique, yet the challenges we face at each stage tend to have things in common. Disruption and change, which feel discomforting, are also times when we are more amenable to reflection. This can lead to reaching out for help or leading our lives more resourcefully.

References

1 Bridges W (1980) *Transitions: making sense of life's changes*. Addison-Wesley, New York.
2 Erikson E (1950) *Childhood and Society*. Vintage, London.
3 Olds S *Her First Week* From *The Wellspring*. The Random House Group, London.
4 Winnicott D (1965) *The Family and Individual Development*. Tavistock Publications, London.
5 Mitchell A (1997) *Beattie is Three* From *Heart on the Left*. Bloodaxe Books, London.
6 Day Lewis C (1992) *Walking Away – for Sean* From *The Complete Poems*. The Random House Group, London.
7 Feinstein E *Getting Older* From *Collected Poems and Translations*. Carcanet Press Ltd, Manchester.
8 Jung CG (1931) *The Stages of Life: collected works 8*. Routledge & Kegan Paul, London.
9 Hill S (1997) *Being Fifty*. Bloodaxe Books, London.
10 Joseph J (1992) *Warning*. Bloodaxe Books, London.

CHAPTER 4

Spirituality, nature and religion

To see a world in a grain of sand
And a heaven in a wild flower,
Hold infinity in the palm of your hand,
And eternity in an hour.
(William Blake, *Auguries of Innocence*, c. 1803)

If 20 people were asked, 'What do you understand by the word spiritual or spirituality?' there would probably be 20 different responses. They might range from 'being religious', 'in touch with God', 'in touch with your deepest self', 'feeling at one with the universe', 'connected to nature', 'a different sense of time' or 'a sense of mystery, awe or wonder'.

In this chapter I shall explore the spiritual dimension of human experience, its importance in forming part of an integrated personality and where it might feature in psychotherapy and counselling. I shall also examine the central role poetry and other creative arts play in communicating this experience.

Can spirituality be defined?

All the definitions I have suggested seem to be an attempt to put into words a feeling or a sense that is almost indescribable and yet is recognisable. Spirit literally means the 'vital principle', which perhaps links it to a sense of energy. Additionally, the various responses imply a depth of experience and a sense of wholeness. Feltham and Dryden (1993) include in their definition of spirituality 'a concern for a quality or domain of life beyond the self centred, the materialistic and the culture bound'.[1] If, as I have suggested, a spiritual sense is important in achieving an integrated personality, it follows that constant superficiality, dealing only with the surface of life, and a fragmented personality are likely to lead to a deep sense of unease. This can be at an individual or societal level.

One difference in approach towards the subject of spirituality is whether we are talking about the experience as encompassing a relationship with an external being or power such as God or a god, or whether we feel that spiritual experience is within human boundaries. Both views will be explored in this chapter. Brian Thorne (1993), describing its place in a therapeutic relationship, says:

> It is important to separate the notion of spirituality from a belief structure which posits the existence of God or an elaborated system of religious dogma. As far as the counsellor is concerned, spirituality has relevance primarily because it concerns the nature of the self and the relationship between counsellor and client.[2]

Much artistic endeavour seeks to communicate this profound sense of connectedness either to the universe or to a transcendental power. Sacred music, religious paintings, cathedrals, mosques and temples are creative expressions of a spiritual force rooted in a religious perspective. In the West, as religion has declined in importance, much of the expression of these sublime feelings has centred on the natural world. For many people the night sky, the wildness of a forest, the sound and energy of the ocean, watching a hawk soar upwards on an air current or the beauty of a single flower are experiences that connect them to something within yet outside themselves. Sometimes it is a response to life or death, or a deep encounter with another human being, which elicits a spiritual feeling. Some people link these experiences with religion: others feel that organised religion attempts to hijack experiences that are wholly within the human domain.

Some examples

Two poems follow that express joy, awe and a wonder in nature. One clearly links these feelings with a concept of God, the creator: the other does not.

> i thank You God for most this amazing
> day:for the leaping greenly spirits of trees
> and a blue true dream of sky;and for everything
> which is natural which is infinite which is yes
>
> (i who have died am alive again today,
> and this is the sun's birthday;this is the birth
> day of life and of love and wings:and of the gay
> great happening illimitably earth)
>
> how should tasting touching hearing seeing
> breathing any–lifted from the no
> of all nothing–human merely being
> doubt unimaginable You?
>
> (now the ears of my ears awake and
> now the eyes of my eyes are opened)[3]
> (E E Cummings)

April Rise

If ever I saw blessing in the air
I see it now in this still early day
Where lemon-green the vaporous morning drips
Wet sunlight on the powder of my eye.

Blown bubble-film of blue, the sky wraps round
Weeds of warm light whose every root and rod
Splutters with soapy green, and all the world
Sweats with the bead of summer in its bud.

If ever I heard blessing it is there
Where birds in trees that shoals and shadows are
Splash with their hidden wings and drops of sound
Break on my ears their crests of throbbing air.

Pure in the haze the emerald sun dilates,
The lips of sparrows milk the mossy stones,
While white as water by the lake a girl
Swims her green hand among the gathered swans.

Now, as the almond burns its smoking wick,
Dropping small flames to light the candled grass;
Now, as my low blood scales its second chance,
If ever world were blessed, now it is.[4]
(Laurie Lee)

The E E Cummings poem addresses God directly as creator of 'the leaping greenly spirits of trees' and seems to be saying that through the beauty of nature he gains a heightened sensibility:

(now the ears of my ears awake and
now the eyes of my eyes are opened)

Laurie Lee makes no reference to God though he does use the word *blessing*. I take the line 'Now, as my low blood scales its second chance' to mean that the natural world – the sounds, sights and smells – has rekindled his zest for life. This is one of numerous examples where a poet uses images from nature as inspiration and as a means of reconnecting with a higher range of feelings.

Counselling and therapy

Does this have a relationship with what happens in counselling and therapy? I think it bears a very close relationship. People often seek therapy because they feel they have lost touch with a life force or libido within themselves: they might say they feel flat, unmotivated, directionless or impotent. Individuals may not put into words that they are seeking inspiration, or want to get in touch with more profound feelings or rediscover an essence of life they feel is lacking. Sometimes they come with a problem with work or with a problematic relationship. It gradually emerges that behind the initial problem lies a sense of emptiness or aridity.

It is not easy to articulate such feelings, which may not seem catastrophic, like a death or a divorce, but which leave people feeling restless and dissatisfied with life. Metaphors and poetic imagery are often the bridge both in describing this monochrome world and then in reconnecting to a richer one.

Which psychological theories give importance to ideas of spirituality? Perhaps it would be easier to start with therapies that do not. Behaviourism and cognitive behavioural therapy emphasise faulty learned behaviour, or the development of unrealistic and damaging belief systems about oneself and other people, as the primary cause of emotional distress. Examining and replacing those behaviours and beliefs is the focus of this kind of therapy. It is not so much that they discount spiritual or sublime experiences as that they are not within the province of their work.

Jung and spirituality

Various psychological thinkers split with Freud because of what they saw as his emphasis on the pathological aspects of human behaviour and his absence of a loftier vision of human potential. Jung wrote of Freud:

> For all his interest in other fields, he constantly had the clinical picture of neurosis before his mind's eye . Anyone who has this picture before him always sees the flaw in everything, and however much he may struggle against it, he must always point out what this daemonically obsessive picture compels him to see: the weak spot, the unadmitted wish, the hidden resentment, the secret, illegitimate fulfilment of a wish distorted by the censor. Nowhere does he break through to a vision of the helpful, healing powers that would let the unconscious be of some benefit to the patient.[5]

Jung, who remained a Christian all his life, had a wide interest in all aspects of religion, including eastern religions and mysticism, whereas Freud was an atheist and regarded faith in an external being as evidence of continued dependence on a parental figure. Jung placed a high value on spirituality and regarded the exploration of it with his patients as a central part of therapy, saying that a religious attitude was an element in psychic life whose importance could hardly be over-rated. He used the word *numinous*, first coined by Rudolf Otto in 1917, which he described as:

A dynamic agency or effect not caused by an arbitrary act of the will. On the contrary, it seizes and controls the human subject, who is always rather its victim than its creator. The numinosum is either a quality belonging to a visible object or the influence of an invisible presence that causes a peculiar alteration of consciousness.[6]

Apart from a personal unconscious Jung believed that humans had a collective unconscious, something each of us is born into, which contains shared images and mythologies. These could be experienced through dreams and fantasies, and were a source of creativity and energy. This is why he referred to the healing power of the unconscious, which could be of benefit to the individual.

The idea of the transpersonal

Jung was the first therapist to use the word *transpersonal* and for him it meant roughly the same as the collective unconscious as opposed to the personal unconscious. For other therapists a closer description would be spirituality. John Rowan's (1993) book, *The Transpersonal*, gives a detailed description of what is meant by the transpersonal, the practitioners most associated with its ideas and some of the techniques used, and he says:

> The process of therapy may be defined in this frame of reference as one of expanding consciousness, allowing the client to discover and integrate the inner wellsprings of transpersonal experience.[7]

A transpersonal therapist does not necessarily work in a completely different way from other therapists and will work with many of the same issues as other counsellors. However, she will be someone who has worked at depth with her own spiritual journey and believes that the pursuit of spiritual experience is one that leads to psychological healing. Therapeutic work is likely to focus on helping a client remove barriers to spiritual awareness. Techniques that might be used include active imagination, a conscious use of images and symbols, or meditation. All of these techniques have the same purpose: to awaken the individual to the profound and creative forces that he or she already has within.

To work in this way does not involve inventing something new: rather, it is about discovering what is already there. It echoes Plato's view that all poetry is 'recollection': it awakens what is already there.

Robert Assagioli, an Italian psychiatrist and a contemporary of Jung, is the other therapist most associated with describing and working with the transpersonal element of human personality. He stressed the value to the individual and society in discovering and nurturing a sense of universality and called his approach 'psychosynthesis'. Whitemore (1991) comments:

Working transpersonally goes beyond the boundaries of a client's individuality. It is hard to define the transpersonal Self because it cannot be easily expressed in words or abstract concepts. It is a living experience for which we find metaphors in all cultures: Ulysses' Odyssey – a long journey whose purpose is to find a way home; Dante's Divine Comedy in which Dante eventually reaches heaven, but only after he experiences hell, purgatory and confronts his shadow; the Holy Grail, for which man searches to find the source of life and immortality. There are many stories and many versions of each, yet they have a single common theme: that there is a centre of life, a place where we feel whole and complete, and that this lies within ourselves. The realization of this source is the heart of transpersonal work.[8]

This sense of wholeness, expressed very simply, is at the heart of much of eastern poetry, as this tenth-century Japanese poem shows:

Watching the moon
At dawn,
Solitary, mid-sky,
I knew myself completely:
No part left out.
(Izumi Shikibu)

Maslow, Rogers and the Humanist School

What is referred to as the Humanist School of psychotherapy has much in common with transpersonal ideas. It places a high value on human potential but without the same explicit emphasis on spirituality. The Humanist School of therapy emerged during the middle of the twentieth century. Its main protagonists were Abraham Maslow and Carl Rogers in America. Like Jung, they were dissatisfied with the concept of forming a theory of human behaviour by extrapolating from patients who were manifestly unhappy and disturbed. They felt that psychoanalytic theory neglected the basic psychological drive in human beings to become fulfilled in every part of their lives. They did not deny that repression, a lack of affirmation and a poor self-concept led to deep unhappiness and conflict. However, they preferred to emphasise that, with a supportive psychological climate, people were capable of growth, social harmony, happiness and a realisation of love and creativity. They felt that each human being has an inbuilt drive towards such self-realisation or self-actualisation.

When barriers to this psychological fulfilment are removed Maslow (1954) describes a phenomenon he calls 'peak experiences', which he describes as:

Feelings of limitless horizons opening up to the vision, the feeling of being simultaneously more powerful and also more helpless than one ever was before, the feeling of ecstasy and wonder and awe, the loss of placement in time and space with, finally, the conviction that something extremely important and valuable has happened, so that the subject was to some extent transformed and strengthened even in his daily life by such experiences.[9]

Rowan[7] comments that it is through peak experiences that we get glimpses of the world of soul or spirit.

Rogers (1980), when describing the right psychological climate for humans to fulfil their potential, often drew comparisons with nature, saying, 'My garden supplies the same intriguing question I have been trying to meet all my professional life. What are the effective conditions for growth?'.[10] Throughout his professional life, once his ideas crystallised, Rogers stuck to the simple but powerful belief that people needed to experience congruence (authenticity), acceptance (to be valued for what and who they were) and empathic understanding. He felt this was the soil of life and, just as a plant deprived of light, nutriments and moisture could not prosper, the individual could not flourish without these essential psychological conditions. Therapeutic contact, for Rogers, involved the therapist offering these core conditions to the client.

Poetry and nature

We have seen that, in transpersonal work, images and active imagination are used to help people feel connected to a deeper part of themselves. Imagery, metaphor and evocative sounds – the tools of poetry – are used to achieve the same aim. Poems about nature are by no means the only subject matter, but I have chosen to focus on them because they are used so often and in many different cultures. Nature is often the vehicle a poet uses to express deeply human and spiritual experiences, those described by Maslow's 'peak experiences'.

Much of the poetry of Dylan Thomas reflects these feelings, as this extract from *Fern Hill* shows:

And as I was green and carefree, famous among the barns
About the happy yard and singing as the farm was home,
In the sun that is young once only,
Time let me play and be
Golden in the mercy of his means,
And green and golden I was huntsman and herdsman, the calves
Sang to my horn, the foxes on the hills barked clear and cold,
And the Sabbath rang slowly
In the pebbles of the holy streams.
(Dylan Thomas, *Fern Hill*, 1946)

Thomas uses images from nature: the barking foxes, the pebbles of holy streams, as the means of connecting to a life-affirming energy. This tradition started in English poetry with the Romantic poets. Wordsworth, in particular, felt that a love of nature led to a love of humankind and that humans were at their best when closest to nature. He felt that Man had a bond with nature which he broke at his peril. He put forward a view of nature as the provider of the right psychological climate for human growth and happiness. Over a hundred years later Rogers explored the human qualities necessary for the same outcome.

Not all responses to nature are joyful and life-affirming, however. Sometimes the feelings invoked are ones of fear, destructiveness or insecurity, for example Ted Hughes' poem *Eagle*:

Eagle

Big wings dawns dark.
The Sun is hunting.
Thunder collects, under granite eyebrows.

The horizons are ravenous.
The dark mountain has an electric eye.
The sun lowers its meat-hook.

His spread fingers measure a heaven, then a heaven.
His ancestors worship only him,
And his children's children cry to him alone.

His trapeze is a continent.
The Sun is looking for fuel
With the gaze of a guillotine.

And already the White Hare crouches at the sacrifice,
Already the Fawn stumbles to offer herself up
And the Wolf-Cub weeps to be chosen.

The huddle-shawled lightning-faced warrior
Stamps his shaggy-trousered dance
On an altar of blood.[11]
(Ted Hughes)

The poem evokes images of power and powerlessness, aggressor and victim, using religious language. The imagery is quite disturbing: like many of Hughes' poems it reflects a totally unsentimental view of nature.

Nature as inspiration, as educator, as nurturer, as battlefield. It is as if nature carries our feelings, or we project onto nature certain feelings, often very intense ones. When Keats hears the nightingale he longs to *be* a nightingale, or at least have the qualities of a nightingale because the bird's song is immortal, and because:

Thou wast not born for Death, immortal bird!
No hungry generations tread thee down;
(John Keats, *Ode to a Nightingale*, 1820)

The nightingale's song is a metaphor for freedom, immortality and an escape from worldly anxieties. This illustrates what I said earlier about metaphor being the bridge or conduit from inner to outer experience.

Depression and loss of the natural world

Responding to the richness and variety in nature seems a healthy part of our human experience. Although the environment to which we feel attuned may vary depending on what is familiar to us – desert, ocean, forest or agricultural scene – most people feel a connection to some form of landscape. It also seems inborn: no one has to teach us how to respond. Just watch a one-year-old child placed on a grassy expanse or a sandy beach, or an older child walking through a wood when the wind is tossing the trees around. However, in times of deep crisis, this connection can be lost. This is especially so when people are suffering from depression. Dorothy Rowe (1983), who writes eloquently on the experience of depression, says:

> It is this peculiar isolation which distinguishes depression from common unhappiness. It is not simply loneliness, although in the prison of depression you are pitifully alone. It is an isolation which changes even your perception of your environment. Even objects around you seem further away, although you know it is not so, and while you are aware that the sun is shining and the birds are singing, you know, even more poignantly, that the colour has drained from the sky and the birds are silent.[12]

If we return to the idea of spirit as being 'vital principle' it is evident that, in a severe depression, this is eclipsed by a mood of heaviness, lack of volition, fear and pessimism. It is part of what makes depression a very frightening experience. As Dorothy Rowe says, you know that you are living in a changed world but it is the internal rather than the external world that has changed.

Most of us go through life sustained by a variety of small and important things: sharing a good meal with friends or family; watching a favourite television programme; going for a walk; listening to music; friendship, love, work; creating something or responding to creativity. In depression, whether it is caused by immediate life events or comes out of the blue, none of these props seem to function.

Coleridge, in his poem *Dejection: an Ode*, calls the experience:

A Grief without a pang, void, dark and drear,
A stifling, drowsy, unimpassion'd Grief

That finds no natural outlet
(Samuel Taylor Coleridge, *Dejection: an Ode*, 1802)

Wordsworth expresses something similar in his *Ode. Intimations of Immortality*, which could be described as a meditation on a spiritual crisis concerned with issues of life and of death. He grieves the loss of the intuitive, intense bond with nature that he experienced as a child:

The rainbow comes and goes,
And lovely is the rose,
The moon doth with delight
Look round her when the heavens are bare;
Waters on a starry night
Are beautiful and fair;
The sunshine is a glorious birth;
But yet I know, where'er I go,
That there hath passed away a glory from the earth.
(William Wordsworth, *Ode. Intimations of Immortality*, 1807)

Sharing the painful journey of the experience of depression is often at the core of counselling and therapy. The counsellor may be aware that happier times are ahead, that, to return to Dorothy Rowe's metaphor, 'the colour will return to the sky and the birds will once again sing'. She cannot impose this optimistic view on her client, but can be alongside her client, waiting to validate and share in a restoration of psychological energy. In my experience, there is always a tiny indication that something has shifted and it is often expressed in an ability to respond, even in a small way, to everyday natural things – a flower, a cloud pattern or an animal. Wordsworth's *Ode* ends with recovery, though with a changed vision:

We will grieve not, rather find
Strength in what remains behind.
In the primal sympathy
That having been must ever be.
(William Wordsworth, *Ode. Intimations of Immortality*, 1807)

Many people, including therapists, may be involved in helping someone recover from a depressive episode. Increasingly, creative arts are also acknowledged as having a vital role in enabling people to express the distress they are feeling and explain their feelings to themselves and others.

Anxiety

Anxiety is closer to depression than many people realise, perhaps because our image of them is so different. Depression has the connotation of someone slowed down, pessimistic and heavy, whilst anxiety conjures up a picture of someone overactive, nervous and rushing around. But often, anxiety is a way of warding off feelings of failure, despair and inadequacy, and depressed people are often very anxious underneath the heaviness and lack of will. Both states frequently focus on issues of loss or feared losses.

Many things in life cause people anxiety: exams, a new job, finding a partner, keeping a partner, the fear of separation, actual separation, fear of death and suffering. Over and above this is what has been called 'existential anxiety', which refers to deeper anxieties about our very existence in the world. At the other end of the spectrum is a profound sense of personal security, perhaps a spiritual peacefulness. Most people have experienced a range of these feelings and, understandably, want to feel more of the latter. The point at which people seek counselling or therapy is often when specific or generalised anxiety becomes unbearable. There are two poems, separated by almost 200 years, that express this anxiety with great beauty but also with resolution.

When I Have Fears

When I have fears that I may cease to be
Before my pen has gleaned my teeming brain,
Before high-piled books, in charactery,
Hold like rich garners the full ripened grain;
When I behold, upon the night's starred face,
Huge cloudy symbols of a high romance,
And think that I may never live to trace
Their shadows, with the magic hand of chance;
And when I feel, fair creature of an hour,
That I shall never look upon thee more,
Never have relish in the faery power
Of unreflecting love;–then on the shore
Of the wide world I stand alone, and think
Till love and fame to nothingness do sink.
(John Keats, 1818)

Keats was not indulging in a romantic melodrama when he wrote this poem. He was terminally ill with tuberculosis and involved in an unrequited passion. The poem does not say exactly what makes him look on love and fame as unimportant, but there is a transformation in the poem's last two lines. He finds something greater outside himself with which to identify.

The other poem is by Wendell Berry and starts with the same sense of anxiety:

The Peace of Wild Things

When despair for the world grows in me
And I wake in the night at the least sound
In fear of what my life and my children's lives may be,
I go and lie down where the wood drake
Rests in his beauty on the water, and the great heron feeds.
I come into the peace of wild things
Who do not tax their lives with forethought
Of grief. I come into the presence of still water.
And I feel above me the day-blind stars
waiting for their life. For a time
I rest in the grace of the world, and am free.[13]
(Wendell Berry)

Although this poem uses images of nature – the wood drake, still water and the day-blind stars – I think it is about much more. It suggests that it is the identification of the poet with the characteristics of these objects that moves him from a position of fear to one of inner strength. He derives strength from the birds who do not have to worry about the future, the water that is still, not turbulent, and the stars that will appear once it is dark. This poem evokes for me some of the same sensations as a deeply enriching therapy session where a client moves from a fragmented, anxious state to a calm, integrated resolve. Even the line 'For a time I rest in the grace of the world, and am free' parallels the process of therapy whereby a client is not 'cured' of his anxiety in a single session. Through the continued and deepening therapeutic relationship he begins to feel more confidence in 'the grace of the world'.

Counselling and therapy cannot take away an individual's external problems, but, by freeing the client from destructive anxiety, can help him to access the deeper, more resourceful part of his personality, including his spiritual side.

Freud thought that anxiety was felt in response to shameful or conflicting instincts arising from the unconscious, for example murderous feelings, forbidden sexual desires or the fear of annihilation. He thought that people employ defence mechanisms such as denial or projection to stop them bringing such thoughts to consciousness. During therapy, therapist and patient worked at understanding the use of the defence so that the anxiety could be experienced at a conscious and thus less threatening level. Again, many people find writing a less threatening way of exploring these powerful sensations.

The sense of time

At the beginning of the chapter I said that a 'different sense of time' was one of the ways in which people describe a feeling of spirituality, those moments that T S Eliot, in the *Four Quartets* 'Burnt Norton' written in 1936, describes as 'At the still point of the turning world'. Many people think that, with our modern obsession with rush, living each moment at breakneck speed, under the tyranny of the clock, we become estranged from the ability to 'live in the moment'. The consequence is that the spiritual side of ourselves gets squeezed out. Perhaps it is one reason why Thomas Hardy has once again become a best-selling novelist – because he describes a time when people lived within the rhythms of nature and the seasons. Kathleen Raine explores this in her poem:

I Had Meant to Write

I had meant to write a different poem,
But, pausing for a moment in my unweeded garden,
Noticed, all at once, paradise descending in the morning sun
Filtered through leaves,
Enlightening the meagre London ground, touching with green
Transparency the cells of life.
The blackbird hopped down, robin and sparrow came,
And the thrush, whose nest is hidden
Somewhere, it must be, among invading buildings
Whose walls close in,
But for the garden birds inexhaustible living waters
Fill a stone basin from a garden hose.

I think, it will soon be time
To return to the house, to the day's occupation,
But here, time neither comes nor goes.
The birds do not hurry away, their day
Neither begins nor ends.
Why can I not stay? Why leave
Here, where it is always,
And time leads only away
From this hidden ever-present simple place.[14]
(Kathleen Raine)

Conclusion

This chapter has ranged over a wide spectrum of issues: transpersonal and humanistic approaches to therapy; depression and anxiety; spirituality, nature and the nature of time. We have looked at the way different poets attempt to give words to these experiences. If, at times, it has seemed a confusing journey, it is perhaps because the depth of these experiences makes it difficult to express them in words: they are often 'beyond words'. But, it is in the nature of human beings to go on struggling to communicate the depth and complexity of this experience.

References

1 Feltham C and Dryden W (1993) *Dictionary of Counselling*, Whurr Publishers, London.
2 Thorne B (1993) *Questions and Answers in Counselling in Action*. Sage Publications, London.
3 Cummings EE From *Complete Poems*. WW Norton & Company Ltd, London
4 Lee L *April Rise*. From *Selected Poems*. PFD, London.
5 Jung CG (1939) In memory of Sigmund Freud. In: (2003) *Jung, The Spirit of Man, Art and Literature*. Routledge, London.
6 Jung CG (1937) *Collected Works*, Vol 11. Routledge & Kegan Paul, London.
7 Rowan J (1993) *The Transpersonal*. Brunner Routledge, Hove.
8 Whitemore D (1991) *Psychosynthesis Counselling in Action*. Harper & Row, San Francisco.
9 Maslow AH (1954) *Motivation and Personality*. Harper & Row, San Francisco.
10 Rogers C (1980) *A Way of Being*. Houghton Mifflin, Boston.
11 Hughes T. *Eagle* From *Under the North Star*. Faber & Faber Ltd, London.
12 Rowe D (1983) *Depression, The Way Out of Your Prison*. Routledge, London.
13 Berry W (1968) *The Peace of Wild Things*. From *Collected Poems* 1957–1982. North Point Press.
14 Raine K (2000) *I Had Meant to Write*. From *The Collected Poems of Kathleen Raine*. Golganooza Press, Suffolk.

CHAPTER 5

Attachment and loss

The word 'happiness' would lose its meaning if it were not balanced by sadness.
(CG Jung)

Why do people come to counsellors and psychotherapists? There are many reasons and many narratives – problems with relationships, anxiety, depression, eating too much or too little, loss of a job or problems at work; worries about changes brought about by poor health or disability. Behind many of these stories emerges a sense of loss – the loss of a partner, a beloved child or a parent; the loss of a job, health, role or a future that was once thought secure.

To lose something implies that you once felt you were in possession of it. It also implies that, to come to terms with the experience of that loss, adjustment and change are necessary. The change can be in the way we view ourselves, our role, our daily routine, our behaviour, life without someone who was central to it. It is this sense that the world is no longer how we once perceived it and that, for equilibrium to be re-established, we must go through some upheaval which is at the heart of our distress.

Poetry, so brimming over with expressions about love of various natures – love of a man, love of a woman, a child, a parent, a dog, a landscape – is equally full of expressions about loss, reflecting this cornerstone of human existence. For the paradox is that we cannot be human without needing and seeking out attachment to and love of people, objects, landscape or to a sense of purpose. But, in so doing, we make ourselves vulnerable to their loss. Poets frequently write about these mirror images: love, birth, passion, security and fulfilment, on the one hand; death, parting, love thwarted or curtailed, on the other.

The next two chapters seek to explore this area of human existence. This chapter deals with attachment and the experience of loss. The next is concerned with recovery or 'regeneration'.

Love and attachment

Poets write about love a great deal: therapists appear not to write about it, or at least not romantic love, very much. This is probably because so much of their work is concerned in working with people where love has 'gone wrong' or the object of a person's love is lost. So, perhaps it is not surprising that they are more immersed in looking at the factors that stop people getting satisfaction from loving relationships than they are in extolling the virtues of love. But, it would be a mistake to think that they do not value love, and see it as a prized goal in life. Freud said that the object of human existence was to 'work and to love', while humanist practitioners like Rogers see love as an essential part of our humanity.

It would therefore seem mean-spirited, before going on to explore issues of loss, not to celebrate the other side of the coin – the joy, exultation, fulfilment and satisfaction to be found in the experience of love. It is what many clients are struggling to achieve. Feelings of parental love are found in poems in the section on Transitions and there are poems that express love of nature in the chapter on Spirituality. Below are two poems that celebrate two very different aspects of a love of one person for another.

Sonnets from the Portuguese

How do I love thee? Let me count the ways.
I love thee to the depth and breadth and height
My soul can reach, when feeling out of sight
For the ends of Being and ideal Grace.
I love thee to the level of everyday's
Most quiet need, by sun and candlelight.
I love thee freely, as men strive for Right;
I love thee purely, as they turn from Praise.
I love thee with the passion put to use
In my old griefs, and with my childhood's faith.
I love thee with a love I seemed to lose
With my lost saints, – I love thee with the breath,
Smiles, tears, of all my life! – and, if God choose,
I shall but love thee better after death.
(Elizabeth Barrett Browning, 1850)

Atlas

There is a kind of love called maintenance,
Which stores the WD40 and knows when to use it;

Which checks the insurance, and doesn't forget
The milkman; which remembers to plant bulbs;

Which answers letters; which knows the way
The money goes; which deals with dentists

And Road Fund Tax and meeting trains,
And postcards to the lonely; which upholds

The permanently ricketty elaborate
Structures of living; which is Atlas.

And maintenance is the sensible side of love,
Which knows what time and weather are doing
To my brickwork; insulates my faulty wiring;
Laughs at my dryrotten jokes; remembers
My need for gloss and grouting; which keeps
My suspect edifice upright in air,
As Atlas did the sky.[1]
(Ursula A Fanthorpe)

Here we have two aspects of love – the passionate declaration, where the beloved triggers feelings of the most ideal kind, and the tried and proven 'sensible' love. Many people would argue that the success of a long-term relationship rests in partners' ability to inhabit both worlds, or at least to negotiate some shared view of moving from one to the other. One of the theories of what makes continuity and maintenance of loving relationships possible is 'attachment theory'.

John Bowlby and attachment theory

As was explored in the chapters on transitions in life, psychodynamic theory is rooted in a developmental approach. This posits that the child's relationship with its parents is at the heart of healthy emotional development. John Bowlby, a psychiatrist in the Freudian tradition, developed Freud's ideas of the child–parental bond but with a significantly new perspective. He abandoned the central notion of sexuality as the main instinctual force, and saw instead the attachment bond between child and parent as the 'blueprint' for emotional development. By attachment, he meant the need of the baby, then child, to have a secure, consistent attachment figure from which to explore the world. If people developed anxious or depressed behaviour, he felt that it was more likely to be in response to attachment issues resurfacing.

The two poems I have just quoted above brought to mind one of Bowlby's remarks on attachment:

Many of the most intense emotions arise during the formation, the mainte-nance, the disruption, and renewal of attachment relationships. The formation of a bond is described as falling in love, maintaining a bond as lov-ing someone, and losing a partner as grieving over someone. Similarly, threat of loss arouses anxiety and actual loss gives rise to sorrow; whilst each of these situations is likely to arouse anger.[2]

Bowlby believed that the way we react to loss is likely to be influenced by our experience of earlier losses in life, such as separations, withdrawal of love or disappearance of the 'attachment figure'. He did not believe we could prevent losses occurring but that we would cope with them better if we had not already been subjected to sudden or consistent losses.

Loss as a 'given'

Irvin Yalom, an existential psychotherapist, names one of the 'givens' of human existence the death of oneself and of those we love.[3] The knowledge is there, but it does not always shield us from the ache or pain, shock or feelings of guilt. William Blake encapsulated this existential 'given' when he wrote:

> Man was made for joy and woe;
> And when this we rightly know
> Thro' the world we safely go.
> (William Blake, *Auguries of Innocence*, c. 1803)

It does seem that people who try to shield themselves from the possibility of loss, or think all misfortune is unfair, unkind or punitive; who live their lives with the view that tragedy is something that happens to other people, often are those hit hardest when they themselves inevitably experience a loss. Equally, when someone has experienced a grievous loss, and in time comes to incorporate it into their life's experience, he or she is often in a better place emotionally to face other losses. They are certainly in a much better position to offer emotional support and sustenance to others. Conversely, if a loss is not acknowledged, given voice to, and grieved, it may continue to be active and render the individual fearful of further losses. Much therapeutic work with clients involves helping them complete all that is involved in the process of grieving a loss.

It is not unusual in psychology to regard reactions to loss, whether the loss is through death, separation, abandonment or traumatic change, as having certain things in common. I have heard bereaved people who have found this an unattractive theory. They feel that to suggest death is comparable to the loss of a job or leaving your homeland is to trivialise their experience. It is true that death brings about a finality, in which that loss can never be reversed, yet I believe that to see a link between all attachment and loss makes sense. In other words, the degree of sadness and devastation felt is directly related to the emotional energy that the person has invested in the lost person or object.

If we look at W H Auden's poem, *Twelve Songs IX*, made famous by the film *Four Weddings and a Funeral*, it certainly appears to be written about a death:

> Stop all the clocks, cut off the telephone,
> Prevent the dog from barking with a juicy bone,
> Silence the pianos and with muffled drum
> Bring out the coffin, let the mourners come.
>
> Let aeroplanes circle moaning overhead

Scribbling on the sky the message He Is Dead,
Put crêpe bows round the white necks of the public doves,
Let the traffic policeman wear black cotton gloves.

He was my North, my South, my East and West,
My working week and my Sunday rest,
My noon, my midnight, my talk, my song;
I thought that love would last for ever: I was wrong

The stars are not wanted now; put out every one;
Pack up the moon and dismantle the sun;
Pour away the ocean and sweep up the wood;
For nothing now can ever come to any good.
(W H Auden, *Twelve Songs IX*, 1936)

Many people are strongly drawn to this poem because it portrays the utter devastation, emptiness and despair that can be felt following a death. It describes a
spoiled world, 'For nothing now can ever come to any good'. However, is this
not also the emotion some people feel at the ending of a close relationship? After
reading the poem many times I have sometimes wondered if it represents a
metaphor for all deeply felt losses.

Freud's views on loss

In his essay on *Mourning and Melancholia* (1917) Freud described mourning as
'the reaction to the loss of a loved person, or to the loss of some abstraction which
has taken the place of one, such as one's country, liberty, an ideal'. He continues (my comments in square brackets):

> Reality testing has shown that the loved object no longer exists, and it [the
> ego] proceeds to demand that all libido shall be withdrawn from its attach-
> ments to that object. This demand arouses understandable opposition – it is a
> matter of general observation that people never willingly abandon a libidinal
> position, not even when a substitute is already beckoning to them.

> Each single one of the memories and expectations in which the libido is bound
> to the object is brought up and hypercathected [heightened with emotional
> energy] and detachment of the libido is accomplished in respect of it. Why
> this compromise by which the command of reality is carried out piecemeal
> should be so extraordinarily painful is not at all easy to explain in terms of
> economics. The fact is, however, that when the work of mourning is completed
> the ego becomes free and uninhibited again.[4]

Like much of Freud, there may be phrases and concepts that strike readers as
overly confident or formal. However, I believe that the notion of the psyche

gradually disengaging and withdrawing the energy it has invested in a loved person or object is a valuable one. The individual is thus freed to engage in life again. He also describes well that part of mourning whereby each memory, each expectation is aired 'piecemeal', however painful. This is usually what happens in grief. When poets write about their sadness and grief in separation from the loved object, that is precisely what they are doing – recalling an image, a sound, a taste or another memory.

Stages of loss

Bowlby saw the process of bereavement as echoing that of a child separated from its 'attachment figure' and described different phases of that process:

> He believes the psychological response to the trauma of separation is biologically programmed in the same way that the inflammatory response is an orderly sequence of physiological responses to physical trauma – redness, swelling, heat and pain. The early phases of grief consist of an intense form of separation anxiety. The later phases result from the confusion and misery that arise from the realisation that the secure base to whom the bereaved individual would turn for comfort in distress is the very person who is no longer available.[5]

The four phases of mourning that Bowlby described are:

- numbness
- yearning, searching and anger
- disorganisation and despair
- reorganisation.

This idea of stages has been embraced by other writers on loss and bereavement. Kubler-Ross (1969)[6] called them Denial, Anger, Bargaining, Depression and finally Acceptance, whereas Parkes (1970)[7] calls them Numbness, Pining, Depression and Recovery.

Is this a useful way of looking at loss? Some writers, for example Thompson (2002),[8] have objected to this model, pointing out that it ignores the individuality of the loss, its context and the cultural strengths that different groups can draw on in responding to death. Yet, there is value in looking at loss as a process, even while acknowledging that every loss is unique and people will not necessarily go through each stage or in a particular order.

Poets would be unlikely to be very interested in some linear progression of feelings, yet they constantly write about loss. They are much more likely to write about the essence of any one of the feelings involved in any one of the 'stages of grief'. Let us look at these in more detail.

After great pain, a formal feeling comes.

After great pain, a formal feeling comes.
The Nerves sit ceremonious, like Tombs –
The stiff Heart questions was it He, that bore,
And Yesterday, or Centuries before?
The Feet, mechanical, go round –
Of Ground, or Air, or Ought –
A Wooden way
Regardless grown,
A Quartz contentment, like a stone –
This is the Hour of Lead –
Remembered, if outlived,
As Freezing persons, recollect the Snow –
First – Chill – then Stupor – then the letting go –
(Emily Dickinson, 1862)

Emily Dickinson never uses the word *numbness* yet every image is imbued with it; the nerves like tombs, the stiff heart, the feet mechanically turning, contentment like a stone and the coldness of snow. Yet there is a sense of progression in the last line. The 'letting go' implies to me that this state cannot last for ever. The fact that the poem starts with the word 'After' implies a 'next'.

And of course we know that emotional numbness seldom lasts forever. Bowlby saw the numbness as a protective mechanism, temporarily shielding the individual from the full impact of loss. People describe the news of a sudden death, or the realisation their partner is having an affair, or the time they are called into their manager's office and told they are no longer needed, or a doctor gives news of a serious diagnosis, as shocking and numbing. It is the reason that many people are 'lost for words' or feel 'rooted to the spot' and wish afterwards that they had said more, asked more, protested, expressed love.

Whilst a person is still numb he or she is unlikely to be able to feel any other emotion. Of all the emotions surrounding loss, numbness is the one most likely to be experienced physically, a bodily sensation. An individual certainly needs support at this time, but not counselling. They are dealing with innate, uncontrollable sensations and are unlikely to be able to 'absorb' anything other than warmth and common humanity.

It would be misleading to say that all experience of loss is then followed by anger, but anger is very often associated with loss; anger at the unfairness of the situation, anger at being deserted, anger at the doctor or other professionals who 'should have prevented' the loss; anger at the upheaval the loss has caused. The feeling is often just a sheer irrational anger associated with a loss of the world as the individual knew it. A poem that expresses this jumble of rational and irrational thoughts beautifully is Bill Holm's *The Dead Get By With Everything.*

The Dead Get By With Everything

Who do the dead think they are!
Up and dying in the middle of the night
leaving themselves all over the house,
all over my books, all over my face?
How dare they sit in the front seat of my car
invisible, not wearing their seat belts,
not holding up their end of the conversation,
as I drive down the highway
shaking my fist at the air all the way
to the office where they're not in.
The dead get by with everything.[9]
(Bill Holm)

What appeals to me about this poem is that it expresses the anger in a genuine but ironic way and it also touches on the aspect that Bowlby mentions – pining and searching for the loved one. Many people talk about an intense sensation of the presence of someone who is lost to them, and this poem describes eloquently the intrusiveness and intensity of that presence. In 'not holding up their end of the conversation' he also captures that emerging feeling of emptiness when you lose someone from death or separation. They are no longer there in their familiar setting, giving security and meaning to your day or routine.

A poem that simply dwells on anger is Vasko Popa's *Give Me Back My Rags*:

Give Me Back My Rags

Just come to my mind
My thoughts will scratch out your face

Just come into my sight
My eyes will start snarling at you

Just open your mouth
My silence will smash your jaws

Just remind me of you
My remembering will paw up the ground under your feet

That's what it's come to between us.[10]
(Vasko Popa)

This is an example of what I described as the 'distillation of one emotion' and in many ways it is a bleak, comfortless poem, reflecting a bleak and comfortless state of mind. We can speculate that the poet feels betrayed by his lover, or something that was ideal has been lost to him. If someone stayed for years in this state of mind, they would indeed be stuck in an emotional wasteland. Yet, particularly in marital or couples work, that is often the feeling that comes across even after many years. As Freud expressed it, 'the shadow of the object has fallen across the ego'.

There is a story told of an American Indian man who felt great sorrow and rage after a catastrophe where there was a great injustice. He said to his grandson, 'I feel as if I have two wolves fighting in my heart. One wolf is the vengeful, angry, violent one. The other wolf is the loving, compassionate one'. The grandson asked him, 'Which wolf will win the fight in your heart?' The grandfather answered, 'The one I feed'.

W B Yeats also uses the same word when he says:

We had fed the heart on fantasies,
The heart's grown brutal from the fare;
More substance in our enmities
than in our love; O honey-bees
Come build in the empty house of the stare.
(William Butler Yeats, *Meditations in Time of Civil War*, No. 6, 1928)

Yeats was talking about what he regarded as the savagery and self-delusion of those prosecuting civil war in Ireland. It is an interesting metaphor – the idea of feeding vengeful or self-deluding thoughts. In psychotherapy the therapist may well suggest to the client that he is displacing angry feelings that originate from an earlier time in his life. In cognitive behavioural work the therapist might ask the client to dispute his beliefs: 'Where is the evidence that A has caused B?', 'Could there be a different or more realistic explanation of how B has been caused?'.

Selima Hill wrote a short poem that captures the emptiness and helplessness a sense of absence can engender:

Your Face

I haven't seen your face for so long now
I feel like a small exhausted traveller
who, coming home one evening in late summer
across familiar fields in fine rain,
finds a ruin where her house should be
and no one there to greet her at the gate.[11]
(Selima Hill)

This seems to echo Bowlby's assertion that it isn't just the forming of attachments that is important for a sense of emotional well-being but the maintenance of them. I have heard clients talk of a feeling of being 'marooned' or having 'no moorings' when an attachment figure moves away or becomes emotionally distant. This can be when children leave home or a friend who was a confidante moves away or any situation where something that was secure and taken for granted is no longer so.

Appropriate losses

As stated, the reason why some people object to the idea of 'stages of loss' is that it appears to reduce people to clones, all going through the same process, and that is palpably untrue. No good counsellor would ever listen to a client, mentally ticking off stages of grieving, but she would be aware that grief is a time of great change and adjustment. Many people describe the death of a loved elderly parent or grandparent as a sad but ultimately fulfilling experience. They recognise the end of a life as a natural process and have had the time to prepare themselves for the death. They can dwell on the many happy memories that have been shared, think of the individual's achievements and fulfilment in life and 'let go'. As in Shakespeare's famous speech from *Cymbeline*:

> Fear no more the heat o' the sun,
> Nor the furious winter's rages;
> Thou thy worldly task hast done,
> Home art gone, and ta'en thy wages:
> Golden lads and girls all must,
> As chimney-sweepers, come to dust.
> (*Cymbeline*, 1609, Act IV, Scene 2)

These lines reflect a sense of completion and acceptance of the death. There is also a philosophic acceptance that life itself must end in death, which encompasses an individual but a universal theme. It also has to be acknowledged that some losses involve a great sense of relief because the individual can then let go of a range of negative feelings.

Loss of the future

In contrast, there are deaths and losses that are hard to mourn and accept because they involve loss of the future. It is said that when an old person dies the past is lost, but when a young person dies, the future is lost, not just their future but the future the parents and others close to him or her envisaged. Again, Shakespeare speaks eloquently:

> Death lies upon her like an untimely frost
> Upon the sweetest flower of all the field.
> (*Romeo and Juliet*, 1595, Act IV, Scene 5)

There are other losses of the future that do not involve death but cause a deep sense of emptiness, isolation and despair. These include severe and degenerative illnesses, disability, miscarriage and infertility. This sort of loss can be particularly hard because it is not clear what the loss is exactly: there may be moments of hope which then prove to be empty. The person is uncertain exactly what they are adjusting to. But they know clearly that something very precious, often taken for granted, has vanished. This is an extract from a longer poem dealing with infertility.

IVF

I come home early, feel the pale house close
around me as the pressure of my blood
knocks at my temples, feel it clench me in
its cramping grasp, the fierceness of its quiet
sanctioning the small and listless hope
that I might find it mercifully empty.
Dazed, I turn the taps to fill the empty
tub, and draw the bathroom door to close
behind me. I lie unmoving, feel all hope
leaching from between my legs as blood
tinges the water, staining it the quiet
shade of a winter evening drifting in
on sunset.

Perhaps I wish the petitioning of my blood
for motherhood might falter and fall quiet,
perhaps I wish that we might choose to empty
our lives of disappointment, and of hope,
but wishes founder – we go on living in
the shadow of the cliffs now looming close:

the blood that's thick with traitorous clots of hope;
the quiet knack we've lost, of giving in;
the empty room whose door we cannot close.[12]
(Kona Macphee)

Kona Macphee expresses that painful ambivalence between nourishing a hope, with all the pain of disappointment, and abandoning the hope in order to 'empty our lives of disappointment'. Sometimes, people experiencing strong conflicting emotions can feel they would be better off if there had been a death. I have heard clients whose partners have left them for another say, 'At least if he'd died I would have had my good memories'. Or, watching someone suffer a painful or debilitating illness, long for the finality of death. Whatever the lost hope is, it needs to be acknowledged and grieved before the person can move on.

Conclusion

In this chapter I have looked at some ideas around the issues of loss. In using the words 'move on', I do not wish to imply that it is an easy thing to do. In the following chapter I will explore the way in which both poetry and therapy can help that process.

References

1 Fanthorpe UA *Atlas*. From *Collected Poems 1978–2003*. Peterloo Poets.
2 Bowlby J (1979) *The Making and Breaking of Affectional Bonds*. Routledge, London.
3 Yalom I (1989) *Love's Executioner*. Penguin Books, Harmondsworth.
4 Freud S (1917) *Mourning and Melancholia*. In: Strachey J (ed.) Standard Edition Volume 11. Penguin, Harmondsworth.
5 Holmes J (1993) *John Bowlby and Attachment Theory*. Routledge, London.
6 Kubler-Ross E (1969) *On Death and Dying*. Macmillan, London.
7 Parkes CM (1972) *Bereavement: studies of grief in adult life*. International Universities Press, New York.
8 Thompson N (2002) *Loss and Grief*. Palgrave, Basingstoke.
9 Holm B (1990) *The Dead Get By With Everything*. Milkweed Editions, Minneapolis, USA.
10 Popa V (1997) *Give Me Back My Rags*. From *Collected Poems*. Anvil Press Poetry, London.
11 Hill S (1997) *Your Face* From *Violet*. Bloodaxe Books, London.
12 Macphee K (2004) *IVF*. From *Tails*. Bloodaxe Books, London.

CHAPTER 6

Loss and regeneration

Poets have revealed themselves and have analysed (the human) condition long before human behaviour was conceptualised as a science. The poet entices participation. In effect, he says, 'Here are my sorrows and my joys, my hopes and my fears. It pleases me to share them with you. If you see yourself in the mirror of my art and feel comforted or strengthened, follow me'.
(L Wolberg, 1969)[1]

In the previous chapter I described some of the feelings and thoughts around loss, and illustrated these with poems written on the subject. I also looked at the ideas Freud and Bowlby had brought to bear. In this chapter I shall attempt to look at some aspects of therapeutic work in loss and bereavement whilst continuing to include poems that illuminate this experience.

Tasks of mourning

William Worden (1983) reviews all the different attempts to describe phases of mourning but concludes:

> Although I have no quarrel with Bowlby and Parkes and their schema of phasing, I think the Tasks of Mourning concept which I present is as valid an understanding of the mourning process and much more useful for the clinician. Phases imply a certain passivity, something that the mourner must pass through. Tasks, on the other hand are much more consonant with Freud's concept of grief work and imply that the mourner needs to take action and can do something. Also, this approach implies that mourning can be influenced by intervention from the outside.[2]

Worden describes the tasks of mourning as to:

- accept the reality of the loss
- work through the pain of grief
- adjust to an environment in which the deceased is missing
- emotionally relocate the deceased and move on with life.

As I have already said, it does not take a huge adjustment to formulate these as tasks that befall anyone who has suffered a major loss other than death. A cherished love affair that has ended, severance from a workplace in which individuals have invested a large part of their energies, the loss of health on which one has counted: all require a large amount of re-adjustment and grieving and you only need to substitute the word *person* or *environment* for the *deceased*. All art forms, visual art, music and literature, including poetry, can be a creative force to bring about change and acceptance.

We have looked at poems that express the pain of loss and have explored ways in which they may be beneficial to the person experiencing a loss. To feel someone has shared the same experience as you reduces the feeling of isolation. To understand that strong emotions such as anger, sadness, despair, insecurity and alienation are normal is very helpful. These can all help the tasks of mourning Worden describes – to accept the reality of the loss and to work through the pain of grief. Individuals often find writing their own poems, letters and biographical memories immensely helpful.

After a death, sharing of the experience of loss is often done with family and friends, by swapping memories, looking at old photos, through music, poetry and art, through the passage of time. It is part of life. It is a misleading stereotype to portray grieving people rushing off to counsellors and psychotherapists as if they had no emotional resources of their own. Unfortunately, the myth continues to be promoted by the media. When people come to counselling and explore losses they have experienced it is usually because they either have no empathic person with whom to share their experience or they feel the sympathetic supporter has had enough of them. Sometimes the trauma of loss has been so deeply buried it is almost inaccessible.

Moving on

Many poems that people find inspiring as they cope with grief and loss would fall into the last two of Worden's tasks, those that address moving on. Poets who only deal with the 'dark night of the soul' eventually get a reputation for dreariness and depression. Similarly, therapists who never validate the hopeful, green shoots of recovery in their clients ultimately have a depressing effect on them. For whatever reason, grief and sadness can remain on the therapist's agenda, with no sense of responsibility for helping the person to move on. Of course, it is wrong to encourage someone to move on before they are ready, but hope and recovery should be areas therapists are alive to.

There are two poems I want to look at in connection with the concept of 'emotionally relocating the deceased (or the lost person or object) and moving on with life'. Another phrase that some people find helpful is the concept of 'taking the person with us in a different way'.

Eden Rock

They are waiting for me somewhere beyond Eden Rock
My father, twenty-five in the same suit
Of Genuine Irish Tweed, his terrier Jack
Still two years old and trembling at his feet.

My mother, twenty-three, in a sprigged dress
Drawn at the waist, ribbon in her straw hat,
Has spread the stiff white cloth over the grass.
Her hair, the colour of wheat, takes on the light.

She pours tea from a Thermos, the milk straight
From an old H.P. sauce bottle, a screw
Of paper for a cork, slowly sets out
The same three plates, the tin cups painted blue.

The sky whitens as if lit by three suns.
My mother shades her eyes and looks my way
Over the drifted stream. My father spins
A stone along the water. Leisurely,

They beckon to me from the other bank.
I hear them call, "See where the stream-path is!
Crossing is not as hard as you might think."
I had not thought that it would be like this.[3]
(Charles Causley)

What I find healing about this poem is that it manages to evoke the past, the present and the future. The picnic scene by the stream is clearly a childhood memory – as so often in childhood there is a cloudless sky. The writer is reflecting on it in the present, yet he is contemplating the future when he will join his parents. The stream represents the archetypal transition from life to death and the title, *Eden Rock*, suggests the Garden of Eden. The whole poem is transfused with an acceptance and optimism. It also seems as if the poet is deriving strength from the reassuring tone of his parents, as one imagines he did during their lifetime.

There is a dream-like quality to the poem, and the second one is manifestly a dream. I quoted it in Chapter 1 so I will only reproduce the first verse here:

About ten days or so
After we saw you dead
You came back in a dream.
I'm all right now you said.
(Thom Gunn, *The Reassurance*)

Like the Charles Causley poem, the writer is using the positive, loving memory of the lost one to give him sustenance and encouragement. There is also the interesting idea of a dream being therapeutic in itself. Freud saw dreams as wish fulfilment and a way of dealing with unacceptable drives and conflicts. Jung saw dreams as having a more reparative function, so that the dreamer literally felt refreshed and repaired by the experience of a dream.

In both these examples the poet has relocated the dead person or people. They don't have the rawness and all-consuming passion of W H Auden's poem, *Twelve Songs IX*, nor are they banished to some far-off reach of the mind where they will not cause any pain. They are there as a comforting presence.

A poem that is an antidote to the bitterness of the Vasco Popa poem, quoted in the previous chapter, is one by Derek Walcott. It strikes me as a very warm poem, in which the poet is reclaiming his own identity. Many people describe the experience of recovery from a loss as not only reclaiming their previous self but also discovering strengths of which they were previously unaware.

Love After Love

The time will come
when, with elation,
you will greet yourself arriving
at your own door, in your own mirror,
and each will smile at the other's welcome,

and say, sit here. Eat.
You will love again the stranger who was your self.
Give wine. Give bread. Give back your heart
to itself, to the stranger who has loved you

all your life, whom you ignored
for another, who knows you by heart.
Take down the love letters from the bookshelf,

the photographs, the desperate notes,
peel your own image from the mirror.
Sit. Feast on your life.[4]
(Derek Walcott)

If we are to relocate the lost person in a place that is valued but not so intrusive that it blots out our living relationships, memory is a central concept:

The Darling Letters

Some keep them in shoeboxes away from the light,
sore memories blinking out as the lid lifts,
their own recklessness written all over them. *My own.*

Private jokes, no longer comprehended, pull their punchlines,
fall flat in the gaps between endearments. *What
are you wearing?*

Don't ever change.
They start with *Darling*; end in recriminations,
absence, sense of loss. Even now, the fist's bud flowers
into trembling, the fingers trace each line and see
the future then. *Always.* Nobody burns them,
the *Darling letters*, stiff in their cardboard coffins.

Babykins. We all had strange names
which make us blush, as though we'd murdered
someone under an alias, long ago. *I'll die
without you. Die.* Once in a while, alone,
we take them out to read again, the heart thudding
like a spade on buried bones.[5]
(Carol Ann Duffy)

This poem might be interpreted as featuring someone who is stuck in painful memories, recollections of more passionate times, but I do not read it like that. The poet makes clear that the keeping of treasured bits of our past, even if it is a failed past, is a common phenomenon. 'Some keep them in shoeboxes' and 'We all had strange names which make us blush'. It is like a confessional that can make our secret memories seem more normal and shared. The metaphor of a 'cardboard coffin' and the simile of 'a spade on buried bones' are certainly images of death, but it is a skilful juxtaposition with the 'heart thudding'. I take it to mean that these letters and memories still have a power to stir us, but nonetheless they are now dead to us and firmly in the past. Perhaps it is a more ambivalent resolution than the last two poems, but nevertheless it is a resolution.

Ambivalent feelings

Worden says that 'The most frequent type of relationship that hinders people from adequately grieving is the highly ambivalent one with unexpressed hostility'.[2] That description reminded me of Thomas Hardy and his feelings about the death of his first wife, Emma. Hardy, always a somewhat aloof and reserved man, had courted Emma in the romantic setting of north Cornwall. She was a vicar's daughter and by all accounts their early marriage had been a passionate love match. There followed a long, loveless marriage with Hardy spending most of his time withdrawing to his study and visiting London. When Emma died suddenly without Hardy apparently even having noticed how ill she was, he was stricken with remorse. He visited the scenes of their courtship in Cornwall and wrote a series of lyrically haunting poems:

The Going (extract)

Why did you give no hint that night
That quickly after the morrow's dawn,
And calmly, as if indifferent quite,
You would close your term here, up and be gone,
    Where I could not follow
    With wing of swallow
To gain one glimpse of you ever anon!

Why do you make me leave the house
And think for a breath it is you I see
At the end of the alley of binding boughs
Where so often at dusk you used to be;
    Till in darkening dankness
    The yawning blankness
Of the perspective sickens me!

    You were she who abode
    By those red-veined rocks far West,
You were the swan-necked one who rode
Along the beetling Beeny Crest,
    And, reining nigh me,
    Would muse and eye me,
While Life unrolled us its very best.
(Thomas Hardy)

Hardy wrote several poems with the same subject matter, recalling the early days with Emma, and presumably experienced some kind of catharsis. Sometimes, when clients have not had the chance to say what they wanted to say to the person who has died or disappeared from their life, it is helpful for the therapist to ask, 'What would you like to say to ...'. Gestalt techniques make this even more explicit, sometimes suggesting that the client write a letter to the individual or, in the session, address an empty chair and say the unfinished words. The aim is to bring about a sense of completion to something that is incomplete.

Therapeutic work with grieving clients has no magical formula, although the therapist may use some techniques such as those described above. It involves being an empathic companion, able to tolerate the range of feelings people bring. It involves helping the person to talk about what they have lost – perhaps aided by photos, mementoes and their own writing. It includes encouraging the person to gain the confidence that he or she has the strength to carry on their life without the person or thing that was so special to them. The fact that the therapist is usually separate from the loss itself is helpful. He or she is part of the 'after' rather than the 'before'.

A wider canvas

To be able to see your loss in a wider context of your own life but also life in general needs a perspective of time. But, some people feel strengthened in seeing themselves as part of a greater picture. They draw strength from contemplating the whole history of human experience which is full of sad and difficult things as well as inspiring and affirming ones.

Just to focus on one period of history – the First World War – can demonstrate this. Some of the most sorrowful, angry and haunting poetry came from this time as people struggled to express the enormity of the slaughter, courage and inhumanity that went on.

Anthem for a Doomed Youth

What passing-bells for these who die as cattle?
Only the monstrous anger of the guns,
Only the stuttering rifles' rapid rattle
Can patter out their hasty orisons.
No mockeries now for them; no prayers nor bells,
Nor any voice of mourning save the choirs,
The shrill, demented choirs of wailing shells;
And bugles calling for them from sad shires.

What candles may be held to speed them all?
Not in the hands of boys, but in their eyes
Shall shine the holy glimmers of good-byes.
The pallor of girls' brows shall be their pall;
Their flowers the tenderness of patient minds,
And each slow dusk a drawing down of blinds.
(Wilfred Owen, 1917)

The poetry of the First World War has been so powerful, I think, because, although we are observers, we are still near enough to those terrible events to feel some connection with them. Recently, someone who had to undergo surgery for cancer told me that she had been reading Robert Graves' biography *Goodbye to All That* just before she had been diagnosed. The description of the field stations with young men undergoing surgery with no anaesthetic had shaken and profoundly moved her. She found that their courage gave her strength to face her operation, in modern conditions and with adequate pain relief, with a more resolute attitude.

Siegfried Sassoon, a poet of the First World War, wrote in 1919 one of the most exultant poems ever written. I have always thought of it as a testament to the power of the human spirit to endure and recover.

Everyone Sang

Everyone suddenly burst out singing;
And I was filled with such delight
As prisoned birds must find in freedom
Winging wildly across the white
Orchards and dark-green fields; on; on; and out of sight

Everyone's voice was suddenly lifted,
And beauty came like the setting sun.
My heart was shaken with tears; and horror
Drifted away. O but every one
Was a bird; and the song was wordless; the singing
Will never be done.[6]
(Siegfried Sassoon)

There is something very therapeutic in being able to see ourselves both as individuals but as also part of a society of people. Sheenagh Pugh's poem, sometimes read at international peace conferences, draws together the individual and the public face of hope:

Sometimes

Sometimes things don't go, after all,
from bad to worse. Some years, muscadel
faces down frost; green thrives; the crops don't fail,
sometimes a man aims high, and all goes well.

A people sometimes will step back from war;
elect an honest man; decide they care
enough, that they can't leave some stranger poor.
Some men become what they were born for.

Sometimes our best efforts do not go
amiss; sometimes we do as we meant to.
The sun will sometimes melt a field of sorrow
that seemed hard frozen: may it happen for you.[7]
(Sheenagh Pugh)

Hope is often a feeling that is completely missing when losses occur. It cannot be forced onto someone but will usually come from within when the person is ready. Perhaps supportive friends, family members and therapists have to 'hold the hope' for the individual for a while. I find this view of hope a very perceptive one:

Hope is not optimism. Optimism tends to minimize the tragic sense of life or foster the belief that the remedy to life's ills is simple. The hoping person is fully aware of the harshness and losses of life. Hope is the sense of possibility; in despair and in trouble, it is the sense of a way out and a destiny that goes somewhere, even if not to the specific place one had in mind. [8]

Conclusion

We have looked at a wide range of feelings and thoughts around loss and regeneration. I hope I have never given the impression that people have to recover from grief and loss, nor that it is easy for an individual. Everyone's experience is unique and healing has to take place in its own individual way.

References

1 Wolberg L (1969) Preface. In: Leedy JJ (ed.) *The Use of Poetry in the Treatment of Emotional Disorders*. JB Lippincott, Philadelphia.
2 Worden W (1983) *Grief Counselling and Grief Therapy*. Routledge, London.
3 Causley C *Eden Rock*. From *Collected Poems*. David Higham Associates, London.
4 Walcott D *Love After Love*. From *Collected Poems 1948–1984*. Faber & Faber Ltd, London.
5 Duffy CA *The Darling Letters*. From *The Other Country*. Anvil Press Poetry, London.
6 Sassoon S (1919) *Everyone Sang*. Barbara Levy Literary Agency, London.
7 Pugh S *Sometimes*. From *Selected Poems* (1990). Seren Books.
8 Fairchild RW (1980) *Finding Hope Again: a pastor's guide to counselling depressed persons*. Harper & Row, San Francisco.

CHAPTER 7

Journeys

We don't receive wisdom; we must discover it for ourselves after a journey that no one can take for us or spare us.
(Marcel Proust)

People in all cultures grow up with stories about journeys. They are conveyed in myths, religious stories, legends, fairy tales, novels or contemporary accounts. Because we hear them at such an early age they are often imprinted on our minds before we quite realise their full significance.

Stories about journeys deal with human issues and dilemmas such as heroism, the search for a lost person, object or 'the truth'. They dramatise the process of exposing yourself to experience and being changed by experience, of making choices between one path or another, encountering true and false companions and learning to tell the difference. They explore the role of fate and external interventions, and expose the protagonists to fortune and misfortune.

Often the narrative is described on a rich, imaginative canvas. The story is about an actual journey – Ulysses' 20-year voyage in the Aegean, Orpheus' descent to Hades, Dick Whittington's journey from poor country boy to Lord Mayor of London – but invariably there is an inner journey, an exploration of psychological transformation for the protagonist.

I am referring to the idea of a journey being a metaphor for life or a part of one's life. This chapter explores some literary forms of this metaphor and some therapeutic ideas about 'life's journey', an expression now commonplace in our language. Images from this central metaphor are so deeply embedded in the language that we hardly notice we are using them. Phrases like 'a stormy passage', 'tranquil waters', 'fresh horizons', 'ploughing a hard furrow', 'smooth or steep path' are used in everyday language to describe a psychological state.

A very brief paraphrase of the story of Ulysses, one of the epic journeys in literature, illustrates this convention. After the Trojan War, Ulysses attempts to return, with his men, to his homeland, Ithaca. On the way he faces many setbacks and perils. He is captured by the one-eyed giant, Polyphemus, and he hears the singing of the sirens whose sweet song is a trap to wreck passing mariners. He is enchanted by foreign princesses and is tempted to abandon his goal of returning to his island and family. When he finally reaches Ithaca he finds his position has been usurped and he has to use all his ingenuity to regain his wife and kingdom. By any standards it is a wonderful yarn but the central theme of the story is about keeping faith with your goal and arriving back where you belong.

Links with counselling and psychotherapy

Where do these ideas fit in with counselling and psychotherapy? We do not need to be Ulysses, fighting one-eyed giants or spending 20 years to reach our home, to know about challenges or goals. We do not need to be Dick Whittington to know the sense of discouragement. Each of us is faced with challenges, goals, decisions, true and false experience as we go through life, even if these are not played out on such a public or dramatic stage. It is precisely because we can identify these as human and universal dilemmas that these stories are so popular and enduring.

The question of how to make sense of our experience, our life journey, is central to counselling and therapy. How has my past affected my present and how will it influence my future? People come to therapy wondering if they are seeking the right goals in life, questioning who set those goals or sometimes if they have lost sight of any goals at all. They come wondering about decisions they are making or not making, how life will turn out if they choose one particular path rather than another.

Practitioners using any therapeutic model would be interested in these questions, though they may approach them in different ways. I have chosen to look at cognitive behavioural therapy and transactional analysis in this chapter because I think they have particularly interesting approaches to these issues, but each therapy could make a valuable contribution to the idea of a life journey. Jung, being particularly interested in myths and the commonality of myths in different cultures, constantly emphasised the need for humans to acquire a sense of meaning from life, and saw myths and dreams as guiding that sense of meaning.

Before looking in detail at these ideas about experience, challenge, searching and decision-making, I want to introduce a poem that illustrates much of what this chapter covers. It is by a modern Greek poet, Cavafy, hugely popular still in Greece, but slightly less accessible in translation. In calling the poem *Ithaka*, and thus linking it with Homer's epic poem, I think he meant us to assume that we are responding to a large theme, the whole of life, rather than a small incident.

Ithaka

when you set sail on the voyage to Ithaka
pray that the way be long
full of adventures, full of surprises
surly Poseidon? don't be afraid of him!
mock his anger

the Laestrygonians, the Cyclops
Polyphemus – these you carry within you
your own heart sets them before you
do not fear them

pray that your journey be long
that many a glorious morning
with joy, with delight
you sail into unknown harbours
drop anchor at Phoenician ports
and search out beautiful merchandise
mother-of-pearl and coral
amber and ebony and ivory
and delicate perfumes
yes delicate perfumes and every kind of lovely fabric
pray that you will come to know many cities
many Egyptian cities, learn many things
gather stores of wisdom from the wise

Ithaka will always be in your mind
don't doubt you will arrive there
but do not hurry your journey in the least
pray rather it will last you many years and bring you wealth
and grown old at last drop anchor
in the harbour at Ithaka

arrived there you will find Ithaka
has nothing to offer any longer
but she is no cheat
she has not deceived you
to her you owe your voyage
all your wealth, all your wisdom
and you will know
the meaning of Ithaka.[1]
(C P Cavafy, 1911, translated by Gerard Casey)

This gently didactic poem encourages the reader to adopt a certain approach to
life, lays down some useful lessons if you like. First and foremost it seems to be
saying something about 'expect a good, rich life, full of experience: relish and
embrace experience'. This chimes with Carl Rogers' optimistic view of 'the good
life' and his concept that people should trust their intrinsic experience and their
instinctive valuing process. The poet not only tells us about the riches but, in
the imagery of coral, amber and sensuous perfumes, encourages us to savour
them.

Then, Cavafy has something to say about experience being subjective: it is the way the individual interprets life events that counts. He says, 'Don't fear surly Poseidon or the Cyclops, you won't meet them unless you carry them in your own heart'. This relates very closely with the idea of projection – that we project feared parts of ourselves, like aggression and destructiveness, onto other people, other objects. I do not suppose a writer of Cavafy's depth would literally mean that there are no external objects in life to be feared, or that all you need to get through life is a strong streak of optimism. Rather, he is saying, 'be aware of where those fears come from so that you don't project them onto others'.

Finally, the poem tells us that the pleasure, fulfilment and feeling of achievement are contained in the journey itself, not in arrival at the destination. In fact, the arrival may contain little, the 'promised land' may be poor, but the richness lies in everything you have gained and learned along the way. However, the poet emphasises that it is *essential* to have Ithaca in your mind, to have a concept or a goal towards which you are travelling.

Transactional analysis and the life script

This very wise poem illuminates the importance of the attitude and the values of the individual setting out on his or her life journey. Amongst many interesting concepts in transactional analysis is the one of the 'life script'. The idea of the life script is that each of us creates our life script out of what adults tell us and our own perceptions. Berne (1975), the originator of transactional analysis, described it as 'an unconscious life plan, made in childhood in response to the messages from parents, justified by subsequent events, and culminating in a well defined pay off'.[2] It includes concepts such as whether we are lovable or not, how trustworthy the world is, whether we can expect to get our needs met by asking for things or whether we have to compete and 'do others down' in order to achieve basic requirements. Injunctions like 'You can only rely on yourself' or 'Men only like women who are weak and feminine' or 'It'll end in tears' shape the way we view ourselves and the world. The problem is compounded by the fact that our script works at an unconscious level. It depends on what messages we have received, but also how we have internalised them. This would explain why children in the same family do not necessarily interpret the same message in the same way.

Part of the role of therapy in transactional analysis is to develop an understanding of your life script so that you can change it and develop what Berne called 'autonomy', a capacity for awareness, spontaneity and intimacy. Individuals in this position are likely to trust their own experience, believe in positive and life-affirming relationships and expect to have a measure of control over their lives. Conversely, an individual burdened by his or her life script may hold beliefs that they are unlovable, the world is a dangerous place, the only safe way to get through life is to keep your head down with as low expectations as possible.

These are extremes, and most people have a much more complex life script, but the important point is that individuals are often unaware that they hold these values or self-concepts. At its most destructive, the individual is imbued with pessimism and holds self-defeating and self-limiting views. The work in transactional analysis is to help the person become aware of the script he or she has constructed and encourage and challenge them to change it.

If we return to the Cavafy poem we can see how difficult it would be for someone with a negative and pessimistic life script to embrace the ideas of the poem, the notion of having lofty goals, of relishing experience, of savouring life. They would probably say something like, 'That's all very well for other people. My experience has taught me that life isn't like that'. What they are often unable to acknowledge is that it is not experience *per se* that has taught them, but the attitudes they have brought to their experience.

Before moving on to a closer look at goals in life I want to introduce a poem that deals with a transitional point in life's journey. Seamus Heaney's poem skilfully blends an *actual* journey, that of a plane flight, with the metaphorical journey of the beginning of his marriage. The feeling of having to trust in something potentially quite risky, but also exciting, is beautifully conveyed.

Honeymoon Flight

Below, the patchwork earth, dark hems of hedge,
The long grey tapes of road that bind and loose
Villages and fields in casual marriage:
We bank above the small lough and farmhouse.

And the sure green world goes topsy-turvy
As we climb out of our familiar landscape.
The engine noises change. You look at me.
The coast line slips away beneath the wing-tip.

And launched right off the earth by force of fire,
We hang, miraculous, above the water,
Dependent on the invisible air
To keep us airborne and to bring us further.

Ahead of us the sky's a geyser now.
A calm voice talks of cloud yet we feel lost.
Air-pockets jolt our fears and down we go.
Travellers, at this point, can only trust.[3]
(Seamus Heaney)

The idea of goals

Is it important to have a goal or goals in life, destinations to which you are travelling? The word itself can have a somewhat 'driven' tone and resonate too closely with ideas of ambition, targets or 'management speak'. I think if we re-define goals in terms of things we want to do in life, experiences we want to have, places – actual or spiritual – that we want to inhabit or visit, the concept becomes more flexible. Perhaps the idea of 'goals' becomes so oppressive or unobtainable to some people that they lose themselves in alcohol or drugs.

One of the issues that frequently comes up in counselling and therapy is whether the 'life journey' is too challenging or not challenging enough. Clients present themselves stressed, tired, with a thousand goals they have to achieve, yet get no enjoyment from the process of any of them. They often start by des-cribing their life as one they have to lead, and say they have no choices. Money, demands of children, lifestyle or duty are the sole determinants of how they live. It is always interesting to explore who it is that is setting these goals and how these relate to the life journey they would ideally like, before they can start making changes.

Research into factors that enable people with drug or alcohol problems to change their behaviour indicates that people most likely to be able to make those changes are those who can envisage themselves without their depend-ent habit. In other words, they can almost 'feel themselves into' what it would be like to be free of the dependency. They have a conviction that it is worth going through the struggle of giving up something that has become a neces-sary part of their lives. Similarly, people who want to change the direction their life is taking often need a picture or an image of how their life could be differ-ent if their goals were different. All creative art can be a conduit into an alternative vision.

Two completely contrasting poems that express something about journeys and aspirations follow.

The Lake Isle of Innisfree

I will arise and go now, and go to Innisfree,
And a small cabin build there, of clay and wattles made;
Nine bean rows will I have there, a hive for the honey bee,
And live alone in the bee-loud glade.

And I shall have some peace there, for peace comes dropping slow,
Dropping from the veils of the morning to where the cricket sings;
There midnight's all a glimmer, and noon a purple glow,
And evening full of the linnet's wings.

I will arise and go now, for always night and day
I hear lake water lapping with low sounds by the shore;
While I stand on the roadway, or on the pavements grey,
I hear it in the deep heart's core.
(William Butler Yeats)

From a Railway Carriage

Faster than fairies, faster than witches,
Bridges and houses, hedges and ditches;
And charging along like troops in a battle,
All through the meadows the horses and cattle:
All of the sights of the hill and the plain
Fly as thick as driving rain;
And ever again, in the wink of an eye,
Painted stations whistle by.

Here is a child who clambers and scrambles,
All by himself and gathering brambles;
Here is a tramp who stands and gazes;
And there is the green for stringing the daisies!
Here is a cart run away in the road
Lumping along with man and load;
And here is a mill and there is a river:
Each a glimpse and gone for ever!
(Robert Louis Stevenson, 1885)

The reason I chose these two poems is that they speak to two opposite needs that may occur at any point of someone's life. Yeats' poem, so beautiful in expressing the desire for peace and solitude, for rebuilding bonds with nature, has deep resonance for the individual whose life is spiralling out of control from the pressures of too many challenges or too many of the wrong kind. Just reading this poem, with its long, unhurried lines, has a calming effect, helping the person experience a slower, simpler world and maybe pointing to what is wrong with his or her current lifestyle. It does not seem important whether the person would in reality want to go and live in that isolated way: rather, it is something about regaining contact with a purer, less cluttered part of oneself. There is also a strong affirming tone to the poem in the opening, 'I will arise'. There is nothing about 'I would like to' or 'I dream of.'!

The Robert Louis Stevenson poem, also about a journey, comes from his collection *A Child's Garden of Verses* and holds great appeal for adults as well as children. It conjures up the excitement of a journey and gets its effect by the speedy rhythm that imitates the rhythm of the train. Sometimes when clients come to counselling they are bored, listless, burnt out or dissatisfied with the direction life is taking them. They need to rediscover a sense of excitement and vitality about their lives. There is a curious parallel process here. This poem has energy and vitality in its metre and imagery. It is also a poem that many people have heard and enjoyed as a child, so in a secondary way it can reconnect them to a time when they felt freer, had dreams and limitless horizons.

Making choices

Apart from making decisions about what values, goals and aspirations we adopt in life (and indeed whether it is really us who has made these decisions or simply absorbed them from our parents and upbringing), we also have to make choices as to how to reach those goals. One of the basic tenets of existential philosophy is that, as humans, we are 'condemned to be free', and have to take responsibility for the choices we make. Yet, making choices can be excruciatingly difficult, because we then have to let go of certain possibilities. I cannot think of a poem that expresses this dilemma better than Robert Frost's *The Road Not Taken*:

> *The Road Not Taken*
>
> Two roads diverged in a yellow wood,
> And sorry I could not travel both
> And be one traveller, long I stood
> And looked down one as far as I could
> To where it bent in the undergrowth;
>
> Then took the other, as just as fair,
> And having perhaps the better claim,
> Because it was grassy and wanted wear;
> Though as for that the passing there
> Had worn them really about the same,
>
> And both that morning equally lay
> In leaves no step had trodden black.
> Oh, I kept the first for another day!
> Yet knowing how way leads on to way,
> I doubted if I should ever come back.
>
> I shall be telling this with a sigh
> Somewhere ages and ages hence:
> Two roads diverged in a wood, and I –
> I took the one less travelled by,
> And that has made all the difference.[5]
> (Robert Frost)

This poem seems to illustrate perfectly the fact that we do have to make choices in life even though, to do so, we have to give up certain options. It also says something about the arbitrariness of some choices in life: we could choose one path or another, but having done so, it is likely to set our life in a particular direction from which it is difficult to return. It also seems to be saying that both paths were attractive but the choice he made that day 'has made all the difference'.

Some people in therapy find choices excruciatingly difficult to make and will do anything to avoid making one. Yalom (1989) makes a valuable point when he says that what is really at stake is not so much knowing what you want as letting go of the other options. If you go down Path A you cannot go down Path B or Path C:

> Other patients cannot decide. Though they know exactly what they want and what they must do, they cannot act and, instead, pace tormentedly before the door of decision. Decision invariably involves renunciation: for every yes there must be a no, each decision eliminating or killing other options.[6]

Most therapists, regardless of which model of therapy they are trained in, would claim that part of their work is to help clients explore the blocks to decision-making, examine the choices in front of them, look at their hopes and anxieties, and then come to some point of resolution. An approach that I think is particularly useful in this respect is cognitive behavioural therapy and its close companion rational emotive therapy. These are both therapies that focus on clients' beliefs about themselves and the outside world.

Cognitive behavioural therapy

Cognitive behavioural therapists believe that emotional disturbance is a result of negative and unrealistic thinking, and that by changing this negative and unrealistic thinking, psychological distress can be reduced. Unlike psychodynamic therapists, they are not particularly concerned with exploring the origin of such beliefs: rather, therapists work with their clients to look at how unrealistic beliefs are affecting their mood and behaviour in the current situation.

Thus, they believe that it is not so much experience itself that forms an individual's mood or behaviour, but how he or she interprets that experience. So, for example, a man who has had one failed relationship may think, 'Well, that relationship didn't work out, it obviously failed because I'm not attractive enough to keep my partner, I'm probably going to fail in all future relationships, so best keep away from women'. This particular belief pattern, described by Beck (1976), is called a 'chain of inference'[7], the person inferring one thing from another with no concrete evidence. In this example the man has not only made an inference about his current relationship, but about all future relationships, which then affects decisions in his life. Gilbert (1992) writes that 'usually a subsequent inference is more global, extreme and emotionally laden'.[8]

A cognitive behavioural therapist would work with her client to make him aware of how he was generalising from one relationship to an entire evaluation of himself. She would get him to dispute or question his beliefs and produce evidence to support such a negative way of thinking, and then see if he could substitute these beliefs with more realistic ones. Another concept from cognitive behavioural therapy is the notion that irrational beliefs lead to self-defeating beliefs. Trower et al.[9] quote Ellis and Bernard,[10] who suggested that three particularly self-defeating beliefs are:

- I am worthless because ...
- It is awful that ...
- I can't stand it that ...

If we think of these beliefs in terms of making choices we can see that if a client believes 'It would be awful or catastrophic if this course of action didn't work out', he is going to find it difficult to make a decision with any risk of failure attached. Choices will always be confined to very safe options and the person may become frustrated and depressed at the limits that they have set on their life. Sometimes these restrictions are projected onto other people: 'I would like to apply for a job in Canada but my mother's health doesn't allow me to'.

Cognitive behavioural therapists do not believe that just by changing anxious, depressed and pessimistic thinking into positive thinking all problems are solved. The emphasis is on seeing if beliefs could be more realistic and in helping the person to become aware of the effect on mood of negative thoughts. In the example given it might indeed be that the person made a conscious decision that he wanted to offer his mother support, but the challenging belief would focus on whether there were any other reasons why he felt unable to move.

A sense of vision

Having dealt with some of the issues that affect our journey, like choices and decisions, interpreting experience, whether we have goals that are right for us, I want to return to the idea of an 'Ithaca', a vision in life. In the twenty-first century, we are understandably wary of the word because recent human history has been set in a catastrophic direction by the 'vision' of leaders such as Hitler, Stalin and Pol Pot. Current political language, which often uses the word, is so stale and duplicitous that it is, with a few exceptions, hardly a source of inspiration.

Yet, as humans, we need an individual and maybe a shared vision if we are to lead complete lives. Individually, as we meet the 'triumphs and disasters' of life, we often have to reshape our vision, but it is still important to have one. Stories, dramas, poetry as well as other art forms can help forge that vision but, even more importantly, keep it alive. A very simple poem concludes this chapter. It was written by Raymond Carver shortly before his death from cancer aged 50.

Late Fragment

And did you get what
you wanted from this life, even so?
I did.
And what did you want?
To call myself beloved, to feel myself
beloved on the earth.[11]
(Raymond Carver)

References

1 Cavafy CP (1911) *Ithaka.* Translated by Gerard Casey (1990) from Echoes, Rigby and Lewis, Crawley.
2 Berne E (1975) *What Do You Say After You Say Hello?* Corgi, London.
3 Heaney S *Honeymoon Flight.* From *The Death of a Naturalist.* Faber & Faber Ltd, London.
4 Yeats WB (1893) *The Lake Isle of Innisfree.* From *The Collected Poems of WB Yeats,* Macmillan, London.
5 Frost R (1916) *The Road Not Taken.* From *The Poetry of Robert Frost.* Jonathan Cape.
6 Yalom I (1989) *Love's Executioner.* Penguin Books, Harmondsworth.
7 Beck AT (1976) *Cognitive Therapy and the Emotional Disorders.* New American Library, New York.
8 Gilbert P (1992) *Counselling for Depression.* Sage Publications, London.
9 Trower P, Casey A and Dryden W (1988) *Cognitive Behavioural Counselling in Action.* Sage Publications, London.
10 Ellis A and Bernard ME (1985) What is rational emotive therapy? In: Ellis A and Bernard ME *Clinical Applications of Rational-Emotive Therapy.* Plenum, New York.
11 Carver R *Late Fragment.* From *All of Us.* The Harvill Press.

PART 2

Introduction

We now move on to the part of the book that is concerned with ways in which poetry can be used with clients, individually or in group settings. The emphasis inevitably moves from one where the individual is *responding* to poetry and other literature to one where he or she is *creating* it. The two are not separate entities, however. Reading and hearing poetry is often a stimulus for writing and this in turn can lead the individual back to reading more widely.

As with art and music therapy, the use of literature as a therapeutic tool has grown over the last ten to fifteen years. There are literary therapists, facilitators and creative writers (there is no agreed name for the role) working in many settings – in hospitals, hospices, mental health settings, schools, residential homes and prisons. This part of the book gives an insight into some of the work that is going on but it is by no means a comprehensive account. In particular, I am aware that, for reasons of space, it has not been possible to do justice to the excellent work that is being done in mental health settings and in prisons. Miriam Halahmy, Claire Williamson and Graham Hartill, who have contributed individual chapters on working with groups, working with young people and working with elderly people, all bring a vitality in describing their work – it becomes easy to picture what such sessions are like.

In 1996 Lapidus (Literary Arts in Personal Development) was established to help foster networking amongst interested people, sharing of information and development of education and research projects and programmes. Lapidus collaborates closely with the National Association for Poetry Therapy, an equivalent organisation in the United States of America. Celia Hunt, at the University of Sussex, has pioneered an MA programme in creative writing and personal development, part of the aim being to equip trainees to use creative writing as a therapeutic tool with individuals and groups. Other courses are being developed, and it is likely that, in the near future, a professional qualification will be formalised, similar to that of an art therapist.

As a counsellor and a tutor I find myself increasingly integrating literature and ideas about metaphor and the imagination into my practice. They have always been there in the background and it has been a gradual process to allow them a more central place. I have been guided by 'what works' and realise that I have often been pushing at an open door. There is a hunger in many people to be in touch with the creative part of themselves and to use all of their resources, including their imagination.

I am deeply appreciative of all the people who have allowed us to use their work in the following chapters. In every case permission has been sought and the individual has decided the way in which their work is acknowledged or whether they would prefer to remain anonymous.

CHAPTER 8

Poetry in individual counselling and therapy

The meeting of two personalities is like the contact of two chemical substances: if there is any reaction, both are transformed.
(CG Jung)

The use of poetry and other literary forms can be a valuable enhancement to the therapeutic process. I say 'enhancement' because, from the outset, I need to make it clear that it cannot take precedence over the actual relationship between counsellor and client. The title of this chapter might summon up a vision of the counsellor solemnly handing out a poem at the end of a session, like a religious tract, implying, 'Read this, it will improve your mood; it will illuminate the way ahead'. Obviously, bringing poetry or poetic language into therapy is a much more subtle affair.

Therapists vary in the degree to which they are attuned to language – images, metaphors and rhythms – but, just as it is possible to train yourself to remember more of your dreams by techniques such as keeping a dream diary or trying to recall them as soon as you wake up, so it is possible to become more aware of the language you and your clients are using to communicate. This chapter explores some of the ways of bringing poetry into therapy:

- the therapist's attunement to language
- clients' own creative work
- exploring published poetry and other literature with a client.

The therapist's attunement to language

Language is only one of the forms of communication that goes on within a coun-selling session. Tone of voice, facial expression and body posture are also clues as to how someone is feeling. But language, 'the talking cure', is certainly central to the process. Just as in poetry something profound is often conveyed via a simile or a metaphor, so too in therapy, the deepest feelings are often conveyed in that medium. Siegelman (1990) says that metaphors 'speaking from the unconscious of the client to the unconscious of the therapist can communicate before they are fully understood'.[1]

Wendy Lynch (2001) outlined four principles concerning metaphor in relation to working with clients:[2]

- that metaphor operates in the realms of the pre-conscious and this can apply to both client and therapist
- that a metaphor enriches and provides a key to understanding a client's narrative construction of his or her experience
- that metaphor can lead to a change in the way in which the client sees the world
- that a counsellor who adopts an open attitude to metaphor by allowing, resonating and fostering it will enhance communication, create a sense of discovery and excitement and a greater willingness on the part of the client to self-disclose.

An example from my practice illustrates these points. I worked with a client for several months. Her mood was flat and lifeless: she described herself as having no feelings and said she was just going through the motions of getting up, going to work, cooking a meal, watching television and going to bed. She did not look forward to anything and had no plans for the future. She told me that she had split up from her boyfriend, a man that everyone had thought she would marry. She could not explain the decision, she just did not feel she could make that commitment. In the third session she told me that, a few weeks after this separation, she had gone out with some friends, got drunk and ended up sleeping with a total stranger. In the morning she felt completely numb and horrified at what she had done. She said, 'I could have been a bloody prostitute. My father would be horrified: he used to call me "petal", now I feel dirty and used'.

I said that it sounded as if she felt the petals had dropped off the flower. Did she feel that somehow she would have dropped in her father's estimation if he knew what had happened? She replied, 'Yes, he was very ambitious for me: sometimes it felt like being in a hot house – he was always wanting me to achieve. He boasted to his friends about how clever or beautiful I was. I was like his specimen rose, which was going to win a prize.' For a fleeting second the words of Blake's poem, 'Oh rose thou art sick' came into my mind, with the last line 'and thy crimson joy doth destroy'.

'What does it feel like to be a specimen rose?' I said, and she replied, 'Too prim and too cultivated'. I asked her what sort of flowers she liked: if she had a garden, what would she plant in it? She replied she would like things like hollyhocks and primroses that just came up every year and looked after themselves. 'Ones that are a bit more resilient than a specimen rose, and a bit more natural?', I suggested.

In several subsequent sessions we worked together, looking at just how much she had internalised her father's need for her to be 'perfect'. The client came to feel that she had ended the relationship with her boyfriend because somehow she had sensed that her father felt he wasn't 'good enough' for her. We often came back to the imagery of flowers; the stiff, formal, cultivated ones, often artificially forced and produced, in contrast to wild and prolific flowers that simply bloomed where they wanted to and multiplied easily and naturally. She gradually moved to being easier on herself and accepting that you can make mistakes but it need not be catastrophic. She realised that she did not have to fulfil all her father's expectations; but, equally, acknowledged that there were many times when basking in his praise had been a great prize. In Rogers' terms she had become 'estranged from her authentic self' and there was something about the imagery of flowers that made it easier for her to struggle to express how she would like to be.

To return to Siegelman's remark about a metaphor 'speaking from the unconscious of the client to the unconscious of the therapist',[1] the fact that this client immediately connected her 'dirty' action in a one-night stand with her father's calling her 'petal' set up a sense in me of something contaminated, and I wanted to communicate back to her in the image she had begun. It then seemed to resonate with her because she went on to use more similes from the world of plants. This approach seems to bear out Angus and Rennie's (1988) study that demonstrated the benefits that arise when the therapist enters the client's world through metaphor.[3] These authors compared situations when therapists collaborated or did not collaborate when the client used metaphorical language. They found that where therapist and client 'co-elaborated the meaning of the metaphor' there was a greater willingness on the part of the client to self-disclose. This led to a sense of discovery and excitement.

An example of the difference could be illustrated as follows. Supposing a client says, 'I feel my life is spinning out of control. Every minute there are ten things I should be doing. When I go to bed at night all the emails I haven't replied to go churning around in my head'. The therapist could respond by saying, 'You sound as if you're constantly on edge and someone else is dictating the pace'. Or, she could say, 'That sensation of spinning. I sense that it's making you giddy, so much so that even at night, when you want to rest, it's like being in a state of perpetual motion'. It is not that one response is right and the other wrong, it is just that the second response is more sensitive to the language the client has used and leaves more room for self-exploration.

Pitfalls

Siegelman, who recommends the therapist to 'resonate and foster the metaphor', also warns against overdoing the technique and being overzealous in this way of working. If a client senses that every time he uses a metaphor like 'a mountain to climb' or 'stormy waters' or 'the Garden of Eden', the therapist is going to pounce on it and elaborate, he will probably do one of two things. He will either start to feel that the therapist is more in love with language then she is interested in helping him. Or, client and therapist will collude in focusing purely on language and a lot of real feelings and thoughts will be lost or ignored. Something similar can happen with the use of dream material in therapy. If a client senses that the therapist is primarily interested in dreams, he may bring these as the focus of the therapy, leaving out important things that are happening in his current life.

There is also a distinction between a 'live' and a 'dead' metaphor. A dead metaphor, roughly, is one that has been so overused that it enters the language as a figure of speech and to many people hardly evokes the original image. Examples would be 'dead as a doornail' or 'happy as Larry'. Live metaphors are ones that are fresh and still evoke the image that is portrayed. There is no absolute distinction because everyone's exposure to language is different. A client once told me that his wife had said to him, 'Are you a man or a mouse?'. I had never heard this expression and, for me, it conjured up a powerful image of masculinity versus timidity. But for him it was a commonplace expression and did not resonate particularly strongly.

Clients' own creative work

Many people write, paint or engage in creative activities when they feel sad, troubled or in conflict. One of the strengths of writing poetry is that it can be undertaken almost anywhere, needs no equipment other than pen and paper, and can be of any length. For clients in counselling and therapy, or attending a healthcare setting, it can also be done between sessions: this helps people extend the time they are spending in therapeutic activity beyond the actual meeting between therapist and client, and provides a 'holding' sense of continuity.

The benefits of expressing yourself through poetry can be enormous and include the cathartic value of getting down on paper what was previously in your mind. Feelings can be expressed and validated. When an individual's thoughts are very chaotic and confused, seeing them written down brings a sense of coherence. Re-reading thoughts and feelings expressed earlier can help someone see a sense of movement and progression. Finally, there is the sheer sense of pride and achievement in expressing yourself in a creative way.

Bolton (2004) stresses that the focus of therapeutic writing needs to be on the *processes* of writing rather than on the products, and says, 'To be therapeutic, the initial stages of writing need to be encouraged to be personal, private, free from criticism, free from the constraints of grammar, syntax and form, free from any notion of audience other than the writer and possibly the therapist or another reader'.[4] It is unlikely that a therapist would make any comment of this kind, but perhaps she needs to clearly spell out to a client that all these

considerations are unimportant. If the suggestion to write comes from the therapist it is a good idea to let the client know that he is completely free to share any
work with the therapist or just keep it for his own private use. For one person
the thought of another reading their work is inhibiting, for another it is encouraging, as if they carry the image of an understanding friend in their
consciousness.

Examples

A client who was going through great emotional pain and devastation after the
death of her brother through cancer wrote a number of poems at that period.
When she reflected on them, some time later, she realised that the form as well
as the content helped her communicate her feelings. She also realised that she
needed a different form of poem to express a different aspect of her grief:

The Evening Swim

An evening swim like any other it seemed,
The low sun, the undulating dance
Of waves, turning to gold in its soft beams,
Ripples caressed into a rhythmic trance.

One was swimming already without looking back,
Cut his own furrow, forging his path to the sun
The watchers stumbled, eager to follow his track,
Stopped short at the shock of the water, and one by one

Looked out again to the swimmer, afloat on the ocean;
Rings and spirals of fire, unfolding and folding,
Buoyed the dark head up, and bobbed with its motion,
Spread counterpane of gold thread, sea-mountains moulding.

They drew back slowly, silent and chilled to the bone,
As the swimmer slipped on through the glitter and sparkle, alone.
(Hermione)

The client wrote, 'The first poems I wrote after my brother's death were rather
carefully worked out, to fit standard poetic forms like a sonnet or a ballad. Following a conventional scheme made me think more clearly about exactly what
it was that I felt – it didn't make me distort my feelings to fit the form, as you
might think. When I wrote *The Evening Swim* I could not believe that my brother
had died, and so I was looking for an image of a movement that was irrevers-
ible. At the same time I wanted it to show his courage. I also saw that I needed to
think of some comfort in the middle of the violent tearing away that death seems
to be, comfort for me, I suppose, but written as if it were comfort for him:

"undulating", "caressed", "counterpane". The pain of the watchers comes in at the eighth line, where the sonnet form dictates a break in the thought: "shock of the water".

'It made me tremendously sad to write this poem. It was very hard to return to it and improve it, because of the feelings involved and because, if I finished it, it would show clearly that he was dead and would never return. At the same time it helped because the sadness was making something beautiful, not just wearing me out.'

The client also wrote poems that were written more spontaneously, quickly and without revision. This is an extract from one:

Why I am angry that Ben is dead

Why am I angry that Ben is dead?
I'm angry because it is not fair
Because he was a good man
Because he loved Mozart
Because he taught his wife to change a tap washer
Because he loved his grandchildren
Because he laughed at Dennis Norden
Because he made a radio when he was thirteen
Because he kept his mouth open and his head on one side
Because he invented things made out of coathangers
Because I wish he had never gone.
And because I am afraid he will never go;
Because as long as I am alive
He ought to be alive as well;
Because he did everything to save himself
And still could not stop himself from spilling;
Because I am closer to him in his death
Than ever I could be in his life.
(Hermione)

About this poem, she said, 'I found writing poems like this a relief because I could express the more discreditable feelings that come when someone dies: the resentment, the wish that their memory would leave you in peace'.

Another client, working through painful issues of abuse in her childhood, searched for a way of integrating this experience into her adult self, and found writing about it as 'one self to another' a form of healing:

Frozen Peas

Hello little girl with sad brown eyes.
Constant chatting hiding deep sighs.

Hello cuts, welts and bruises,
Sore places from abusers.
Hello little girl with so much to give,
Who would give anything just to live.
Will you let me take your tiny hand,
I promise I will understand.
Will you let me hold you, for the child that you were,
Let me deal with and worry, with what may occur.
Will you let me cry tears for what should have been,
Will you let me love you whatever you've seen?
Your memories are as fresh as frozen peas,
Can I help you to learn you don't have to please?
Let me love you, and hold you, and tell you I'm there,
For all that we've been through, in all that we share.
Let us hold hands together and walk away from past strife,
Let us gently take steps through the rest of our life.
Let our footprints be left for all who can see,
So we can remember when you became me.

A third example is of a client who had been through a severe depression, which was beginning to lift. Through the depression he had experienced his body as heavy, leaden, and static. He arrived with a poem that he read:

Lungs lunge
Ribs uncage
Arms pump
Heart thumps
Feet run
Hands create
Head's higher
Future's brighter

This client wanted both to rejoice in the improvement he felt, which he could best describe through bodily sensations, and also to share the sense of release with someone who had been through this dark period of his life with him.

Therapist's role

Therapists vary in how explicit they are in the way they work with poetry and other literary work with their clients. In some cases it might be responding to and appreciating creative work their clients bring. Some therapists specifically describe themselves as 'poetry therapists' and structure the time with their clients, spending roughly the first half of the session talking about feelings, issues and goals, and half the session focused on poetry, either the client's work or work he or the therapist introduces.

'Poetry writing can enable an effective process of self-communication. It can feel dangerous, just as any effective therapeutic process is experienced as teetering between the destructive and the healing.'[5] The therapist needs to be aware that anyone sharing their creative work is taking a risk. They risk getting in touch with feelings of which they may not be fully aware, they then may fear being judged for having those feelings, thoughts or perceptions. They may also fear judgement of the merit of the work itself.

Assuming the risk is taken, the rewards can be considerable. Once trust is established, creative work can be a very revealing focus with which client and counsellor can work. It could be perceived as intimidating if the therapist were to pore over every word her client has written, but to focus on a detail or to ask a client to say more about a person, an event or a memory can be very therapeutic. Omissions are also revealing. One young client I worked with wrote a poem about his entire family, mother, brothers, sisters, grandparents and pets, and left out any mention of his father.

Exploring published poetry with clients

Increasingly, counsellors and therapists are extending areas of contact with clients, and they might suggest a book for the client to read or take the initiative by introducing a poem and seeking a reaction from the client.

The therapist might say something like, 'How do you respond to this poem? It seems to express some of the feelings or thoughts you were talking about'. Many of the poems I used in Part 1 of this book would be appropriate for use in this way. For instance, a client struggling with feelings of anger or disbelief about a death might respond to the poem by Bill Holm, *Who Do the Dead Think They Are*? Equally, the poem by C Day Lewis, *Walking Away*, can resonate strongly with parents struggling with issues of separation from their children.

Obviously, it is the client's and not the therapist's reactions that are important. As Mazza (2003) points out, a poem can be a springboard for the client to talk about his feelings, goals or values.[6] Sometimes the client responds to the whole poem, sometimes a particular line or image hits home. Poetry is especially valuable when clients are having difficulty connecting with their experience, for example an unexpected death or a rather unspecified anxiety state.

Mazza (2003) quotes a poem by Stephen Crane, *If I Should Cast Off This Tattered Coat*, as having an 'open-ended message':

If I Should Cast Off This Tattered Coat

If I should cast off this tattered coat,
And go free into the mighty sky:
If I should find nothing there

But a vast blue,
Echoless, ignorant –
What then?
(Stephen Crane)

I can see several different interpretations to this poem and it is one that you could respond to in different ways at different times, depending on your mood. It seems to be a poem that explores the grandeur of the universe and the issue of taking risks: to question the purpose of existence, and to ask whether there is anything there at the end of the journey. It challenges the reader to ask, 'What would happen if I made a great leap of faith?'.

This raises the question as to where a poem can take someone emotionally and cognitively. One person might see this as a very liberating poem that enables them to see that they will not achieve any of their dreams unless they are prepared to 'cast off' some of their familiar security. For someone else, it could connect with a deep sense of anxiety about there being no boundary, no absolutes in their life. It could increase anxiety. This shows that, just as in the more conventional 'talking' therapy, the therapist needs to be aware of the effect a poem, a suggestion or an interpretation might provoke. I would not avoid using this poem because of the risk of increasing anxiety, although I would think carefully about the timing and its suitability.

Conclusion

Jung was the first therapist who specifically suggested to his patients that they paint or write as part of their treatment. Supporting and encouraging clients to develop the creative part of themselves is, for me, an important part of therapy.

References

1 Siegelman E (1990) *Metaphor and Meaning in Psychotherapy*. Guilford Press, New York.
2 Lynch W (2001) One client – many stories. Dissertation, University of Manchester.
3 Angus L and Rennie D (1988) Therapist participation in metaphor generation: collaborative and non-collaborative styles. *Psychotherapy*. **25**.
4 Bolton G (2004) Introduction. In: Bolton G, Howlett S, Lago C and Wright JK (eds) *Writing Cures*. Brunner-Routledge, Hove.
5 Bolton G and Latham J (2004) Every poem breaks a silence. In: Bolton G, Howlett S, Lago C and Wright JK (eds) *Writing Cures*. Brunner-Routledge, Hove.
6 Mazza N (2003) *Poetry Therapy: theory and practice*. Brunner-Routledge, Hove.

CHAPTER 9

Running creative writing groups

Miriam Halahmy

Don't tell me the moon is shining: show me the glint of light on broken glass.
(Anton Chekov)

Introduction

Creative writing groups have become very popular and widespread in the past ten years. Interest in writing varies from budding novelists to those who want to explore areas of their personal lives. One young man in a group for the homeless explained to me that writing is the only thing that stops him from screaming out loud in the street. All writers have to be prepared for the fact that feelings and issues that they thought were buried, or did not even know existed, may surface on the page. Managing those feelings in groups, created in different settings and with different types of participants, is an essential part of running a creative writing group.

An artist friend of mine claims that all paintings are self-portraits. I believe equally that all writing is about the self. When people join my groups and say that they have never written before and have no idea where to start, my response is that all writing lies within the subconscious. My job is to facilitate the mining of this rich vein and help to raise to the surface the nuggets they want to explore.

Facilitators of creative writing groups may be trained therapists, published writers, qualified teachers, or perhaps none of these. Currently there are no recognized qualifications for the facilitators of groups in this field. I come from a teaching background and I am a published writer. I have therefore brought these two fields of interest together in the facilitation of creative writing groups in different settings.

Setting up a creative writing group

Creative writing groups form in different settings for different purposes. I have run groups at evening institutes, in settings for the homeless, for writers' projects and in my own home. Sometimes I initiate the setting up of a group and this may involve advertising and charging fees; sometimes I am invited to set up a group by a host institution. One group I run is for 'prime timers' in a private gym. The participants are all aged over 55, we meet each week in the crèche and have published two pamphlets of work.

When forming a group it is important to agree whether this will be an open or closed group. For some purposes, for example in a mental health setting, the host institution may agree with the facilitator a specific group size, for a specific number of weeks. Alternatively, the group may be open to all comers at all times. In the homeless settings I have worked in, participants come and go, sometimes throughout the sessions, and it is therefore very difficult to build a stable group. Facilitators need to have a flexible approach to setting up groups, which will accommodate the interests and needs of the participants, the aims of the host institution where involved and the vagaries of the physical environment available.

The role of the facilitator

The role of the facilitator is to establish a welcoming and enabling atmosphere where trust and confidence can develop and all the participants can have a good experience. One key is to learn names quickly and to greet each participant on arrival by name. The facilitator also needs to demonstrate that she is organised and efficient, conducting the necessary business of the group without fuss. The first session is therefore very important in establishing the ambience and direction the group will take, with the facilitator establishing clear and well-prepared leadership.

My preferred method for opening a group is to introduce myself, giving my background as an experienced teacher and workshop facilitator and a published writer. This information demonstrates to the participants that I have the background to run a creative writing group and helps to engender a sense of trust.

Firm boundaries need to be established at the first session with any group. All groups need boundaries, and it would be a mistake to assume that adult groups are able to keep within unspoken boundaries. When boundaries are not set and maintained, irritations and complaints arise quickly. Quite recently someone in my Prime Time group commented that she really appreciated how I kept the group members in order and did not let them slide into chatting and drinking coffee!

The facilitator needs to consider which boundaries she would like the group to follow, and then present them to the group for agreement. Boundaries might include:

- starting on time
- finishing on time

- only one person speaks at a time
- silence when someone is reading aloud
- listen and respond to each other with respect
- no 'put-downs'
- it is individual choice whether to read aloud and whether to receive any feedback
- maintaining confidentiality.

Different groups may need different boundaries and flexibility is essential. From time to time boundaries need to be reviewed, and reminders, such as being punctual, may have to be restated. The important thing is that the facilitator establishes and sticks to agreed boundaries from the outset.

Getting started

A good way to start with a new group is with warm-up oral exercises. Participants joining a writing group will have a variety of worries about their writing skills. Older members often say that they were evacuated during the Second World War and their schooling was very interrupted. Many people are worried about spelling and handwriting, and others are concerned about how well they can express themselves in writing.

It is therefore good to start with something everyone can do and everyone can contribute to. One of my favourite 'starters' is to ask each person to give their name and tell one lie about themselves. One round of this usually has everyone laughing at the inventions that emerge – about age, ambitions on the stage and so forth. Another favourite is the 'commonalities game'. Working in pairs, find something in common with your partner, then do this exercise in fours and finally as a whole group. Recently, in my Prime Time group, we discovered that none of us like wearing thongs!

After a few minutes of oral warm-ups everyone has spoken and connected with the other members of the group. It is also useful to go back to these exercises if the group changes, to help to absorb new members.

Brief writing exercises

The facilitator needs to develop a repertoire of brief writing exercises that will take only a few minutes to complete and will help to ease a new group into the process of creative writing. In this way some of the anxieties about producing something 'good' will be reduced. Some people have virtually written nothing since school, several decades ago. Others feel that they are locked into office writing, reeling off long reports, emails and spreadsheets. Brief exercises, some of which can be completed as a whole group, will help to alleviate some of these concerns and pave the way for more in-depth writing later on.

Group work could include brainstorming around one word, for example *love, survival, night*. Write the word in the centre of a whiteboard and ask for associated words or phrases. Then choose a different word or phrase to work on in prose or poetry.

Acrostics can also be a good way to work as a group. An acrostic is a poem in which letters on successive lines spell a word when read downwards. Hence: 'Power Over My Life' would be set out as follows and could form a poem as in the first verse example:

Perhaps I could decide
Only once a week I
Will drink a glass
Even two and never
Risk the nightmares again

Working in pairs or slightly larger groups can also reduce anxiety about writing skills and generate a lot of fun. Simple activities, such as writing one stanza of a poem in pairs, can lead on to more in-depth group work later on. The members of one group I am working with have now decided to write a short play together and have planned the plot and characters and, working in three groups of three, they are writing one scene each.

The facilitator can use these situations to encourage people to work with someone different each time and therefore strengthen the relationships in the group.

Techniques for developing writing skills

In my creative writing groups most people want time to read work from home. Therefore my sessions are a mixture of writing practice in the group and then a workshop session to hear work from home.

Stream of consciousness writing is very popular. I use a range of starters, such as 'I remember when.', 'Today I will.', 'Yesterday.', 'I was walking along the track when.', 'If I were not afraid I would'. I remind participants that they should write for ten minutes without their pen coming off the page and, if they are stuck, they should just copy out the previous sentence or two until their thoughts flow again in any direction. Participants are surprised at how much they write and at the material that surfaces from their subconscious. Often, they find a starting place for a longer piece of writing.

Poems or extracts from classical or contemporary literature are excellent triggers for writing. They helps to broaden the reading experience of participants and provide models for demonstrating good writing, such as dialogue, character, setting and 'showing not telling'.

One poem that I have used very successfully is *What Every Woman Should Carry* by Maura Dooley:

What Every Woman Should Carry

My mother gave me the prayer to Saint Theresa.
I added a used tube ticket, Kleenex,
several Polo mints (furry), a tampon, pesetas,
a florin. Not wishing to be presumptuous,
not trusting you either, a pack of 3.
I have a pen. There is space for my guardian
angel, she has to fold her wings. Passport.
A key. Anguish, at what I said/didn't say
when once you needed/didn't need me. Anadin.
A credit card. His face the last time,
my impatience, my useless youth.
That empty sack, my heart. A box of matches.[1]
(Maura Dooley)

This poem evokes a wide range of responses from participants. Some write poems about themselves. Others are interested in writing as someone completely different. One homeless writer wrote 'What every soldier should carry' and included:

Bravery because they've got to put their lives on the line
and Jesus in their heart because he always knows what to do.

In contrast, a man, writing as a woman, wrote:

red lippy for the face I want to make up.

This is a poem that can both explore the internal world of the writer and allow the writer to step into the imagined world of another.

Extracts from novels, both contemporary and classical, have the dual purpose of demonstrating a technique and introducing participants to writers they may not have heard of. Many go on to buy and read the books. Sharing books is an essential and very stimulating part of a writing group and participants soon find that they are interpreting the texts they read in very different ways.

Carmella has attended my Prime Time group for several years. She writes, 'For me writing is cathartic, it helps me come to terms with certain issues. It is also great fun. I just love creating stories with romantic sexual innuendoes'. Writing also allows her to explore her family relationships. This is a sonnet she wrote about her son, who is schizophrenic:

Sonnet to my Son

The tot, tot of the bike at the back door.

A young man with a helmet, a son I adore.
His eyes when smiling make me feel my best
This is because his demons are at rest.
The torment ever ready to jeer
My heart aches, when I see his gait full of fear.
Tea, biscuits, racking my brain to do my best,
Quiet words, listening, I suggest, tell the bastards to piss off in jest
With pill bring deep slumber, they're gone without a trace
He fights a war but doesn't cry aloud.
I shout, 'Son, I love you and I am so proud.'
Thank God I am alive to bring him so far,
To carry him through when the door is no longer ajar,
My spirit will guide him to travel far.
(Carmella)

The fascination for me in running creative writing groups, in any setting, is the variety of responses to the triggers I offer for writing. My aim is not therapy as I am not a trained therapist. The challenge for the group facilitator is to balance, on one hand, a sensitive and supportive awareness of the possibility of the effect on individuals, and, on the other, providing a stimulating and developing series of workshops.

It is very important for the facilitator to consider carefully any feedback to participants. Sometimes participants simply want to read out their work, and do not want to receive feedback, particularly if their work is very personal. Sometimes they choose not to read back at all. However, in general, everyone in a group is very keen to read their work aloud and to hear comments about it.

Participants want to learn how to improve their writing, and most people in a group are keen to be published at some point. They expect the facilitator to provide points that they can learn from. My approach is to encourage everyone to respond to work read out and to encourage supportive comments, even if they contain an element of criticism. It is essential to create an atmosphere of trust in the group in which everyone feels that they can read out confidently and receive useful feedback that affirms them on their route as developing writers.

The emergence of more deep-seated feelings in a group setting

All writing has the potential to reveal deep-seated emotions and memories. The facilitator needs to ensure that she is always working within the limits of her competence. It would be easy for a writer leading a group to overstep the boundaries and slip into the field of therapy, when deeper themes and feelings begin to emerge. It is also not easy to predict when this might happen as the example below illustrates very clearly.

One exercise I often use with groups is to ask participants, in pairs, to describe to each other a favourite character from a book. One member of a group, Anna, described to me the deep effect this simple exercise had on her. The only character that came to Anna's mind was 'Little Red Riding Hood'. However, she realised as she began relating this to her partner that the story was releasing some very deep memories in her. She had emigrated to America with her parents when she was five. Her parents were Holocaust survivors. Little Red Riding Hood was the first children's story she heard in English and the wolf terrified her: 'The wolf brought up for me the fear and horror that my parents carried with them from their experiences, although they never mentioned them. Working with these painful feelings I was amazed that I could write anything'.

For Anna, joining a writing group, even though not specifically set up as a therapeutic group, allowed her to explore her feelings in writing, at her own pace: 'All the strange feelings of insecurity and fear of being an immigrant in a new country came up for me, painful scary feelings I felt as a young child. When I came home from the writing group I shared those feelings with my husband and daughter. I was quite upset and they were very supportive. In the next class we were given the theme Yesterday and I wrote this poem'.

Yesterday

Five years old
Frightened and confused I walk to school
I want to be home with Mum and baby sister
Where safety is
My class is big
Teacher fierce but she likes me
I feel scared
This is the USA
They do not speak Yiddish
English is a foreign language
For those who don't belong
I colour a circus picture
A pink, purple, smiling trapeze girl winks at me
A golden yellow lion roars out of the page

Thirty years later
I colour a Farm picture with my young son
We make animal sounds Ba Ba, Moo Moo
While the green, yellow, blues and reds dance off the page
I watch the delight on my son's face
I belong.
(Anna)

What is the role of the facilitator, who is not a therapist, in a situation where the participant begins to reveal very deep personal parts of herself and may even begin to cry?

Partly, Anna answers this question herself: 'When the group members saw me crying they were very supportive and said it was all right, I didn't need to read it. But for me the healing was in being able to cry and read, and share the poem with everyone'.

As a facilitator, I feel that my role is to allow the space for such feelings to emerge, and to listen and to validate that the writing has led to the emergence of such deep feelings. However, it is then important to bring closure to that participant, by gently moving on to the next contributor and making it clear that it is not my role to open up a session of group therapy. As I am not a therapist this would be little more than pseudo-therapy and therefore quite dangerous. In addition, although I would not actively discourage strong emotions such as crying, equally, I do not want to give too great an emphasis in this direction, in order that the group does not change direction completely. My aim is always to maintain the focus of creative writing as the chief purpose of the group.

Another quite simple writing starter, using the poem *A Kite for Michael and Christopher* by Seamus Heaney, and a suggestion to write about childhood games, evoked a very strong response from Ruth, a member of my Prime Time group. She was often lonely as a child:

> I had two imaginary friends. They lived in a small cupboard in my room to be summoned in times of loneliness and stress. The centre of my world was my Nanny, who arrived when I was three months old and stayed for 11 years. I owe her everything and, without her, I doubt I would have survived. When I was 11 my father left home to live in Paris, leaving me with my beautiful, alcoholic, neurotic mother and childhood came to an abrupt end.
> (Ruth)

Much of Ruth's early writings in the group, whatever our starting point, explored her difficult childhood, often ending in tears as she read her work out. She says: 'Writing in a group is great fun and it is a privilege to hear others' thoughts and hopes and expectations put on the page'. It is clear that, for Ruth, writing and sharing these feelings has been very affirming.

Working with a specific group: an arts project for the homeless

In this particular setting I have a two-hour weekly slot and many of the participants arrive with sheaves of work they have written whilst sleeping rough or in vulnerable accommodation such as hostels or on a friend's floor. These participants are keen to write so that people can share the thoughts that are running through their heads.

Anthony has just started to write again after a five-year gap. He is working on a rough sleepers' journal. Here is an extract.

Friday Night

There can be no worse fate for a rough sleeper caught in the middle of Leicester Square on a Friday night, within the intermingling crowd who are laughing, shouting, spreading money around and dressed up to the nines, etc., etc.

I listened to my friend as he recounted his story and I could not stop myself laughing as to his circumstances and the way he portrayed his vulnerable position to me. His description of his night in Leicester Square laden down with bags while searching for cardboard and essentials was, for its part, ironic, for maybe a few weeks earlier he had attended Leicester Square in different circumstances walking arm in arm with some pretty woman, not even blinking an eye as a piece of cardboard discarded in the corner comes alive and out pops a head and then a dishevelled body emerges like a caterpillar from a chrysalis.

(Anthony)

Anthony does not write in my sessions, but brings his work for feedback from myself and other participants. He is keen to be published and listens carefully to everyone's comments.

Many of the participants in this project tell me that, for them, writing is a kind of therapy. They find my 'stream of consciousness' starter exercises a very rewarding way of tapping into the thoughts they want to express. J describes writing as 'like climbing out of a murky pool into a marvellous horizon'.

The sessions often take off at breakneck speed, with participants arriving at different times, with poems or short stories they want to read out. Others just want to write, and one woman is working on a children's book that she is also illustrating. Some participants want to talk about their substance abuse or where they will find a bed for the night.

Pulling these mixed demands and interests together, and focusing attention on the purpose of the group, which is to write, is a constant challenge. I always make sure I am prepared with a wide range of triggers for writing, perhaps a set of pictures or a pack of words, maybe a writing frame or a phrase for an acrostic poem. Sometimes we can all focus together and then the group really appreciates the extracts from novels or the poems I bring with me. Many of the participants are very widely read. I have had Nietzsche and Borges quoted at me, along with Orwell, Bob Dylan and Dostoyevsky. We are now at the stage of submitting poems for publication to the newsletter printed by the arts project and this is very affirming for the writers in the group.

Conclusion

All creative writing groups have some therapeutic value as participants begin to explore themselves through writing. The facilitator, who is not a therapist, needs to develop a sensitive awareness of this aspect of the work, while not placing unnecessary emphasis in this direction. My aim, in all my groups, is to provide the best experience of creative writing possible, using high-quality materials, to introduce participants to a range of genres and writers, both classical and modern, and to respond with constructive feedback to the work that they bring to the group. The level of comment and the feedback I offer will be tempered by the individual and the content of their writing. However, no matter what the setting, my approach will be to offer the same high standards of literary input and response in order to give an authentic experience to all the participants.

References

1 Dooley M *What Every Woman Should Carry*. From *Sound Barrier: Poems 1982–2002*. Bloodaxe Books, London.

CHAPTER 10

Poetry in healthcare settings

Health is a state of complete physical, mental and social well-being and not merely the absence of disease or infirmity.
(Preamble to the constitution of the World Health Organization, 1946)

This chapter seeks to describe some of the areas in which successful and enriching work using literature and writing in healthcare settings has occurred or is occurring. It also makes suggestions as to how a facilitator or therapist might proceed, and explores the role of such a facilitator. Attention is also drawn to important practical considerations of working alongside medical staff, and to ethical points when working with patients. Both physical and mental healthcare settings are considered.

Current climate in healthcare

The widespread interest in and use of alternative and complementary medicine, the deployment of counselling and psychotherapy in general practice settings and the use of creative therapies all attest to the gradual move to look at health and illness in a more holistic way. The National Institute for Clinical Excellence (NICE) in its guidelines to doctors 'to improve the treatment and care of people with depression and anxiety'[1] recommends 'that for mild and moderate depression, psychological treatments specifically focused on depression (such as problem-solving therapy, cognitive behaviour therapy and counselling) can be as effective as drug treatments and should be offered as treatment options'.[1]

In 1996 Professor Sir Kenneth Calman, the Chief Medical Officer, Department of Health in England, convened an interdisciplinary meeting of some 40 people to discuss the importance of the humanities in medicine, and how the place of the arts in health and well-being could be emphasised. The meeting led to the Nuffield Trust initiative for the arts and humanities in health and medicine, which included the Windsor Declaration of 1998 for the Arts, Health and Well-being, and the publishing of three reports.[2,3,4] This work has now been taken forward by a joint initiative of the Arts Council, England, and the Department of Health.[5] The Arts Council has reported from its 'Ambitions for the Arts, 2003' that, 'It is our central belief that the arts have the power to transform lives, communities and opportunities for people throughout the country'.[5]

The experience of being a patient

What is it like being a patient in a medical setting? This may seem a naive and over-generalised question but some of the following feelings are likely to be present for anyone admitted to hospital, other healthcare facility or visiting their general practitioner: anxiety, fear of pain, relief, fear of bad news and longing for good news. They include the satisfaction of feeling listened to and being understood, and the frustration of feeling misunderstood. If the reason for the visit is primarily concerned with individuals' mental health they may be worried that they are losing control or 'going mad'.

Added to these concerns is the sense of being an amateur in a world of expertise. The coming together of these two states – anxiety and unfamiliarity – often leads to a great sense of vulnerability. Sometimes this very vulnerability makes patients see medical staff as more powerful or nurturing or withholding than is actually the case.

An art or literary practitioner within a medical setting brings something much more informal and tangential to the environment. Their presence cuts across the medical culture of symptoms, diagnosis and treatment. From the patient's perspective there is no compulsion: you can choose whether to take part. You are no longer defined by your illness but by your interest in the subject and you can be an expert in an environment where you may feel overwhelmed by professionalism. Creating something – a poem, a picture, writing down your thoughts in a journal – strengthens your sense of identity at a time when you may feel you are losing it.

Although the provision of creative arts is not universally available throughout healthcare settings in this country, there is a much greater openness to introducing them alongside conventional medicine. In this chapter it is only possible to give a snapshot of some areas in which literature has been used:

- cancer care
- a spinal injuries unit
- community-based projects
- mental health settings.

Using writing in cancer care

There are many reasons why people with a diagnosis of cancer find creative work helpful. Despite better cure rates, the immediate reaction of most people when they are told they have cancer includes the thought that they might die, or at least that their lives will be radically altered. Just experiencing such thoughts can open up feelings of panic, anxiety, sadness and fears of separation. Equally, the person may find he or she is more focused on what really counts in life, feel very close to special people in his or her life, respond to the natural world in a more intense way and reach out to find meaning in life.

From a practical point of view the individual's life is usually disrupted with hospital visits, admissions, tests, waiting for results and undergoing treatment. This often means that the person spends a lot of time waiting or resting when they would normally be more active. Writing is often a way of filling this space with something personal and constructive, when the alternative is for it to fill up with anxiety.

Many people report that describing fears and anxieties in writing makes them less powerful. Equally, a way of dealing with such feelings can be to focus outwards on to objects in the outside world, in particular the natural world, using all the senses: the beauty of a group of snowdrops; the sound of a hectic city street; an ambulance siren; the smell of orange blossom; the texture of a cat's fur. Dominic McLoughlin, a writer who teaches creative writing in a hospice setting, makes a valuable point when he says, 'Paradoxically, writing gives us the chance to both go towards the self, and to escape from it'.[6]

Below are some examples of writing by people who have had or who are living with cancer. It includes their observations as to how writing was beneficial to them in dealing with the many aspects of their illness.

Recovery

I want to write about fragrant spring days
and going for short walks
because I'm delicate
and need to heal.

What will make me stronger?
What will cause an accumulation of fluids?
What will cause excessive strain?

I want to run and shout
and find the perfect man
to touch my body.

I want someone to know exactly
which secret places
make me moan
and fill with pleasure.

I don't want to compromise
or be careful.
I don't want to hurry.

I am learning patience,
and I feel solid and connected,
knowing I will die
and hoping not for a long time.
Knowing I am flawed
but discovering perfection
at the same time.

Maybe my wounds are perfect
and my disability a gift,
somehow.
And I am patient
and waiting to open the package
to find the sparkling jewels
that really were there all along.
(Wendy Lewis)

Wendy Lewis writes:

'I was diagnosed with a rare type of genital cancer when I was 50, a year after my husband and partner of ten years had left me. I went through surgery, radiation and chemotherapy, and was forced to ask for help and rely on friends in ways that I never thought possible. The poem, *Recovery* was written during that time.

'When I was well enough to go back to work I started going to a writer's group for women with cancer, and it was the first place where I discovered that I could get comfort from other women. I became terribly depressed and wrote some very dark poems. The group heard me and comforted and supported me. I learned that depression and anxiety often follow cancer treatment.

'Now I am feeling quite well again. I sold the house that I owned with my ex-husband and bought a townhouse near my work all on my own. Now my poems are filled with joy as I truly embrace the pleasure of being healthy and the freedom of being on my own.'

Wendy Lewis talks about writing in response to crises in her life, a stimulus for a lot of people to start writing. For people who already write poetry or keep journals, writing is a natural way to respond to a crisis brought about by serious illness. Myra Schneider, a poet who teaches and facilitates creative writing groups, was diagnosed with breast cancer in 2000. Her book chronicles her many varied feelings, thoughts, actions and poems over a two-year period.[7]

One of the techniques she uses is called 'dumping', which she used when she was feeling shocked, frightened or in turmoil. This technique involves sitting down and making a list of all the feelings and thoughts on the individual's mind. She suggests putting each thing that occurs as a single sentence and starting each sentence on a new line. This is an example of the list she made following surgery and before facing a course of chemotherapy:

What's on my Mind

I am terrified of facing chemotherapy.
I am dreading feeling sick and being out of action or partly out of action.
I am afraid of my hair thinning and falling out.
I feel ill just thinking about this treatment.
I feel upset that I have to think about this while I'm recovering from the operation.
I feel overwhelmed that I have so much to contend with.
I feel worried because a tooth has broken and the crown has come off the tooth next to it.
I feel strung up about changing or cancelling work fixtures.
I feel bothered about putting other people out.
I feel ashamed that I swore and threw my clipboard on the floor and made Erwin very tense when the battery ran out while we were listening to his tape recording of the surgeon explaining my results.
I feel it's the last straw to know I might have to undergo radiotherapy too.
I don't want to give up.
I want to retire from Flightways – it would be a relief.
I find it daunting even to think about dealing with this.
I want to focus on doing things day by day.
I want to accept it will take a long time to sort everything out.
I want to put my safety first.
I feel better if I think about what I've already managed to get through and do.
(Myra Schneider)

In commenting on this process she says, 'Again, dumping my jumble of fears and other feelings into my notebook was a tremendous release. Once on paper they stopped going round and round in my head and I began to be more positive and focused'.

Frequently, when reading poems about cancer, or written by people who have cancer, the sense that emerges is that the writer now feels some control over their emotions and their body. This helps restore a sense of safety that the illness has jeopardised.

Work in a spinal unit

A diagnosis of cancer sometimes comes out of the blue, but has often been preceded by some days or weeks of anxiety about the individual's health. Equally, after the diagnosis is made the person may still feel healthy and 'no different' than he or she previously felt. The major source of anxiety is often focused on the future – fear of death or reduced life expectancy or fear of the treatment itself.

Patients admitted to a spinal injury unit after sudden, traumatic injury have had no time to adjust to a catastrophic change in their bodies, their lives or their future. They are placed in a matter of minutes into a situation where the past is irretrievable. They may have been fit, healthy young men or women one day and within a short space of time their whole world is completely changed as they come to terms with paralysis, life in a wheelchair, needing assistance with bodily functions as well as every normal activity. They are also likely to spend a prolonged period in hospital, possibly as long as a year.

Rose Flint, a writer in residence with the Kingfisher Project in the Salisbury area, worked in the spinal unit over a period of seven months. By the time the patients started on the creative writing sessions their medical conditions had largely stabilised and further improvement was unlikely. She describes the initial meeting with the patients, a group of four men and one woman, and her realisation of the enormity of their loss and the struggles still ahead.[8] She wrote, 'I felt as if I had entered another world, somewhere aquatic, alien to me, with a different system of breath and being. I was the stranger, struggling to swim'.

The patients were struggling with feelings of despair, anger, regret and deep feelings of loss. Some expressed a wish that they had died in the accident rather than having to face their present situation and what lay ahead.

The group members, none of whom had written poetry before, expressed a desire to write, although first they wanted to talk. As a first stage it seemed important to help the group members to focus on the here and now, the feelings so palpably in the room. Poems expressing anger, bleakness or feelings of physical humiliation often emerged:

Anger

My anger is dark grey
dark grey
black fog.

My Anger tastes of damp rotten mould,
the odour of second-hand clothes.

My anger is a low rumbling, constant, relentless,
deep in my chest.

My Anger is cold
and sharp as slate.

My Anger fears the light, will stay

nuzzling the dark,
and dream of preventing light's presence
so that dark invades
everywhere.

I meet Anger each morning.
I meet Anger each night.[9]
(James Gregory)

Writing down feelings, sometimes in metaphorical form, as a colour or a texture, allowed them to become externalised and real. Having those feelings then acknowledged and shared within the group gave some recognition to their power.

Another strand that Flint felt was important for the group was some reconnection to the past. 'The past was "Before the accident", somewhere that had become in many ways a place that was now forbidden to these patients. The accident had warped the past.' Memories represented a potential for bringing more emotional pain because they enshrined the loss of the future:

Finding places where someone had been happy and confident – whole – and re-visiting those places *as they had been experienced* became an important part of the work. Slowly, remarks such as *'and I will never do that again'* or *'but I won't ever be able to get there again'* began to change to *'yes, I did that. I am proud of that,'* or *'I'm glad I can remember that'*. Bit by bit it seemed that they were re-assembling all the broken parts of themselves into a new whole.[8]

My Last Walk

That day, in crisp biting weather
with the ground frozen solid
and puddles cracked like plastic on the path,
we'd done half a five-mile circuit
and stood looking out from the high downs
across the level plains of Wiltshire.

Below us the land of patchwork fields
had hardly changed in several hundred years;
we could be looking back in time
into an earlier shire, under the same blue sky.

Haze, a low mist,
then gold
flooding the landscape
distorting the colour, changing soft greens
with the sun's falling.

Time to turn back as we run out of light.

But what I remember so vividly
was that the land was beautiful that day
and I remember my last walk with joy
as something special, without sadness.[10]
(Giles Harding)

Adjustment after a major trauma depends on many things – the hospital environment, support from family and friends, the person's previous outlook on life, the age at which the accident happened and the inner resources the person has to draw from. Having the space, encouragement and support to engage with the whole of your personality through a creative process could be a central thread in the healing.

One of the patients Flint worked with, James Gregory, later published a selection of the group's poems under the title, *My Last Walk*. He writes:

Basically, when you break your back or neck your whole world changes and is turned upside down. There is a lot to come to terms with, a whole grieving process to be endured. It impinges on every little detail of your life, more than most people would ever realise. Prior to my injury I was at the peak of physical fitness and my career had panned out exactly as I had planned it. I was serving as a doctor in a commando unit working in Northern Ireland and, on my first day of a six month tour of duty, I was in a helicopter that crashed and I became instantly paralysed.

There were many therapies in rehabilitation, some of the best therapies for me were those that I did not even realise were helping me to come to terms with what had happened. There are a lot of emotions to wrestle with. There is anger and resentment and reflection on one's whole life, as you prepare to enter into the world again in a completely different shape and form.

The collection of poems is arranged to reflect this progression from bleakness, anger and fear to a sense of a future, however uncertain that future might be. One poem, written just before the patient was discharged from hospital, ends:

At this chrysalis stage who knows if
a hideous bug or a beautiful butterfly lies within?
I have always feared change
yet now I pull it to me like a precious thing.
(Giles Harding)

This progression illustrates some of the points made in Chapter 6. There is a process within the experience of loss that impels people to follow some path of change. Things can never stay the same. The help and support to an individual to express this experience, whether through words, music or art, is the role that a creative therapist seeks to play.

Community settings

The two areas focused on so far concern situations in which people are seriously affected by illness or injury. There are, of course, many other medical and psychological conditions in which people are only affected transiently, or in which they have a long-term but not life-threatening illness. Here, the facility on offer – an art, literature or creative writing group – is situated in a community setting. Below are some examples of projects.

Poems in the waiting room

This is a project devised by Michael Lee, in which pamphlets are available for patients to read and take away from doctors' surgeries. Michael Lee was aware that many people waiting to see their doctor feel anxious and concerned, and the poems are therefore ones that focus on positive topics, such as beauty and transcendence, friends and companionship, care and security. The object is not just to ease the time spent waiting to see a doctor, but also to help people to focus on positive and reassuring images and sounds when dealing with physical and emotional upsets. By 2004 some 1200 waiting rooms were requesting copies of the pamphlets.

Poetry in a general practice surgery

This initiative was set up by a general practitioner with funding from Gloucestershire Adult Continuing Education and Training. The practice funded a poet and workshops were open to both patients and staff. Patients included people suffering from depression, or adjusting to life changes; some had chronic health problems, others were just interested and keen to try a different creative activity:

> Many participants commented on the stress-relieving benefits of taking part and perceived the writing process as therapeutic in some way.
>
> We have to start promoting non-medical therapies for non-medical problems. Every time we prescribe, when there is no true medical problem, we are conspiring to medicalise. Poetry does not cure disease. Neither does diazepam bring back the lover who has left, the mother who has died. Poetry is about something that you didn't quite know was there. It is the process of writing that can surprise you and be uplifting. It makes you feel better.[11]

Art project for patients with ME

This is a project run by Keele University and the Shropshire Wildlife Trust called 'Inner Gardens'. It is aimed at people diagnosed with ME or chronic fatigue syndrome, who 'wish to explore a complementary therapy aimed at increasing interest and energy levels'. It is primarily an art project, but poetry and fairy tales are also used to stimulate the participants' imagination. One participant wrote:

In the early stages of the project the subject matter of our paintings was suggested by the art therapist. We painted the sky at different times of the day, the rainbow, seasonal flowers and plants. While painting, the therapist read a couple of short pieces of poetry. I enjoyed this on many levels. I found it further stimulated my imagination, deepening my appreciation of colour and beauty in nature, and helped me connect on the level of the spirit. Later, I used the material from a simple fairy story as the subject of one of my paintings.

Offering more than one medium for artistic expression can be particularly helpful in enabling people to extend their abilities.

Mental health settings

The link between mental illness, emotional turmoil and writing has often been observed. Poets such as John Clare, Robert Lowell, Sylvia Plath, Anne Sexton and Elizabeth Jennings experienced significant mental health problems and have written about them. This poem by Elizabeth Jennings expresses a mood of great anguish and reflects something of the isolation that is common with severe mental illness:

A Mental Hospital Sitting Room

Utrillo on the wall. A nun is climbing
Steps in Montmartre. We patients sit below.
It does not seem a time for lucid rhyming;
Too much disturbs. It does not seem a time
When anything could fertilize or grow.

It is as if a scream were opened wide,
A mouth demanding everyone to listen.
Too many people cry, too many hide
And stare into themselves. I am afraid.
There are no life-belts here on which to fasten.

The nun is climbing up those steps. The room
Shifts till the dust flies in between our eyes.
The only hope is visitors will come
And talk of other things than our disease.
So much is stagnant and yet nothing dies.[12]
(Elizabeth Jennings)

McLoughlin's remark quoted earlier, that 'writing gives us a chance to both go towards the self, and to escape from it', is particularly apt in mental health settings. Some patients and clients are drawn towards writing down their very intense feelings of isolation, confusion, depersonalisation and anger. Others almost need to avoid inhabiting that space, and find a sense of security in describing familiar objects, the natural world and a happy memory.

A facilitator working in a mental health setting needs to be able to accommodate these two ends of the spectrum. Phillips and colleagues say:

> The vulnerability of group members and their potential unwillingness to share pain and difficulty within the group needs to be remembered and respected. Group members will often resist any direct demands that they should write about themselves, their feelings or experiences, but if they are asked to write about themselves and their memories in an oblique way, they will often share their experiences very generously and openly.[13]

Several facilitators have found that patients or clients often use what they have written to communicate with their therapist or key worker.

Some practical considerations for writers working in a psychiatric hospital setting include the following.

- It is advisable to have two facilitators so that one facilitator can spend time with a distressed or disturbed individual.
- Facilitators need to be realistic about the degree of confidentiality that can be offered. It is probably more appropriate to offer a 'team confidentiality' so that concerns about suicidal or psychotic ideas can be shared with a member of the medical team.
- The medications patients are taking, plus the illness itself, can limit individuals' attention span, so short writing tasks are likely to be more successful.

Survivors' Poetry (www.groups.msn.com/survivorspoetry), set up in 1992, provides workshops, performances, readings, training courses and publications to a wide audience of survivors, healthcare providers and arts professionals. Their anthologies contain many original and highly creative poems.

Role of the facilitator: healthcare settings

At present there is no formal qualification for a 'literature therapist' working in a healthcare setting, unlike an art therapist. Facilitators or tutors usually come from an education, writing or counsellor or therapist background, and they may have experience and training in more than one area. This inevitably influences their approach to the work. The most important thing is that facilitators are clear about their role, both to themselves and to the patients. Most facilitators present what they have to offer as 'a creative writing group' rather than as a therapy group using writing. However, even presented in this way, it is essential for facilitators to be sensitive to and knowledgeable about individual and group dynamics.

The content of the sessions will be determined by the nature of the group, and several writing techniques have been described earlier, in Chapter 9. Reading a poem or a passage from a book is excellent stimulus material. Using a 'spidergram', whereby different images are clumped around a central idea such as 'a room in my home' or 'a place where I feel at peace', can help people to get started.

Because of the nature of illness and treatment, it is unlikely that the same group of people will be present each week, so skill is needed by the facilitator in maintaining a sense of continuity whilst welcoming new people to the group.

Supervision for the facilitator is very important, too. It is vital that the facilitator has somewhere to take the problems and successes that arise from the group and someone with whom she can discuss ideas for helping individual members. Inevitably, being with people with distressing illnesses will also give rise to painful feelings in the facilitator, which she needs to share.

The healthcare setting

Whether the setting is a hospital, hospice, day care or other community facility, good communication with staff is vital. It is discouraging to arrive on a ward to find that the staff have forgotten you are coming and the potential group members are asleep. The best projects are often those where staff themselves get involved in the group, either as co-facilitators or by joining in with the writing task. This spreads enthusiasm and commitment among the staff group. Dominic McLoughlin writes:

> The host organisation has a responsibility to manage the boundaries of the group, for example by making appropriate referrals, ensuring there is a suitable room, providing a member of staff, where needed, to assist clients with special needs, and so on. This support provided at the managerial level is vital to ensure the safety and effectiveness of the writer in health care, thereby enhancing the quality of service that can be offered to their clients.[6]

Ethical considerations on the part of the facilitator include:

- a shared agreement between patients, staff and facilitator over confidentiality within the group
- clarification of links between the facilitator and the host organisation
- permission, usually in writing, for any work to be copied or reproduced
- the facilitator working within her levels of competence; for example, she does not claim to be a therapist if she is not trained, she does not conduct sessions if she is physically or emotionally not capable of doing so.

Evaluation

Of all the settings in which the arts are practised, healthcare is the one that is most likely to be subject to evaluation, ultimately linked to funding. There are plausible physiological reasons for thinking that the calming effect of the literary arts, and especially poetry, is related to an interplay between the left and right cerebral hemispheres of the brain: the left hemisphere analyses and responds to language, the right visualises images and responds to rhythm. This interplay could activate the limbic system at the base of the brain where thought meets emotion.[2]

One qualitative study of comments written spontaneously by 196 members of the general public identified that poetry was helpful with anxiety, depression, bereavement, terminal illness and several other conditions. Seventy-five per cent of respondents reported that reading poetry reduced stress and 66% said that writing poetry had the same calming effect as well as providing an outlet for their emotions; 10% reported that reading poems improved their mood and 13 respondents felt poetry was responsible for their being able to stop antidepressive or tranquilliser medication.[14]

Conclusion

The arts in healthcare is a very wide area and this chapter gives only a taste of the many initiatives in progress. Good physical and mental health are central to our sense of well-being. It is when that sense of well-being is shaken that many people look to other ways of addressing their sense of dis-ease.

References

1 National Institute for Clinical Excellence (2004) *Guidelines to Improve the Treatment and Care of People with Depression and Anxiety* (Available at www.nice.org.uk).
2 Philipp R (1999) Evaluating the arts in health care and mental health promotion – the example of creative writing. In: Haldane D and Loppert S (eds) *The Arts in Health Care: learning from experience*. The King's Fund, London.
3 Philipp R (2002) *Arts, Health and Well-being: from the Windsor 1 Conference to a Nuffield forum for the medical humanities*. The Nuffield Trust.
4 Coates E (2004) *Creative Arts and Humanities in Healthcare: swallows to other continents*. Strategic paper prepared by a collaborative inquiry group. The Nuffield Trust.
5 Arts Council, England, and Department of Health (2004) Cultural medicine: investment in cultural capital for health. *Flux*.
6 McLoughlin D (2004) Any-angled Light: diversity and inclusion through teaching poetry in health and social care. In: Sampson F (ed.) *Creative Writing in Health and Social Care*. Jessica Kingsley, London.
7 Schneider M (2003) *Writing My Way Through Cancer*. Jessica Kingsley, London.
8 Flint R (2003) *Kissing Your Sister: Poetry in the Spinal Unit*. Kingfisher Project, Salisbury District Hospital, Lapidus Issue 5.
9 Gregory J (2004) *Anger*. From *My Last Walk: pictures and poetry by paralysed people*. James Gregory, Tetratastic.
10 Harding G (2004) *My Last Walk* from *My Last Walk: pictures and poetry by paralysed people*. James Gregory, Tetratastic.

11 Wills E and Opher S (2004) Workout with words. *British Journal of General Practice.* February: 156–7.
12 Jennings E *A Mental Hospital Sitting Room.* From *New Collected Poems.* David Higham Associates, London.
13 Phillips D, Linington L and Penman D (1999) *Writing Well: creative writing and mental health.* Jessica Kingsley, London.
14 Philipp R and Robertson I (1996) Poetry helps healing. *Lancet* **347**:

CHAPTER 11

Using poetry with young people: survive and shine!

Claire Williamson

We wake up every morning in an alien environment. Certainly not the environment that man was created in, so to me it is very much a struggle just to be human.
(Lee Stringer)

The above statement was made by author Lee Stringer in a conversation about writing. The climate into which we are born is unavoidable and, for many teenagers, the current climate seems to dictate that if you are not a high-achiever *en route* to celebrity status, it is easy to feel alienated.

I am a writer who has been working with young people since 1996. This work has been executed both independently and with the support of various organisations such as Poetry Slam (an educational performance poetry organisation), WNO MAX (the educational department of Welsh National Opera) and Multi A (a Bristol-based educational arts organisation). I am passionate about working with young people, and about writing. This is bound up with my belief that literature has life-sustaining qualities. It helped me to survive adolescence and has taken me forward to feel as if I can not only survive in the world, but feel a part of it and even shine. As a result of this first-hand experience, I completely trust my tools: poetry, story, song, prose. As the poet Rose Flint says, 'As a writer in healthcare, it has made me really *trust poetry*. What needs to be said, brought from unconscious to the conscious, will be articulated by the voice of poetry if it is allowed freedom'.[1]

I think that *freedom* is the key word here. It is vital that young people feel free to make writing their own; to take possession of the craft and consequently own their feelings and find their voice. This chapter explores some of the processes involved in this journey and will also describe the challenges of introducing poetry to young people. The processes are very much the 'creative process', as described by Silvano Arieti in his book *Creativity: the magic synthesis*.[2] Arieti suggests that the conditions for fostering creativity are:

- aloneness
- inactivity
- day-dreaming
- free-thinking
- being in a state of readiness for recognising similarities
- openness
- the remembrance and inner replays of past conflicts
- discipline.

The aim, potential and pitfalls

The aim, when I work with young people and poetry, is to engage them with creativity, and, specifically, to enage with the creative process to produce an original product. Potential for engagement with writing is huge, as Nicholas Mazza quotes in his book, *Poetry Therapy: theory and practice*: 'Jon Shaw (1981) noted that the adolescent period is one of high creativity'.[3]

'High' creativity means that there is massive potential for young people to engage with the creative process. This potential parallels the prospective formation of a clear and solid sense of self. It is a powerful and yet fragile time in our life. The most effective work with young people can occur if there is an environment of trust, so that they can be 'open' to their own potential. One comment from a young person attending a Poetry Slam workshop articulates, 'As soon as the poets came into the room, I felt that we were friends already and free to write about anything'.

Trust is engendered by treating young people with respect and by being careful to facilitate workshops with clear instructions and accessible language. It is vital that a writing facilitator does not patronise, because the patronising voice is most threatening to the emerging adolescent. An environment of trust allows young people to take risks at this time in their lives when they are incredibly creative. This potential for engagement is counterbalanced by a turbulent life stage. As outlined earlier in Chapter 3, adolescents are experiencing identity formation, rebellion, self-doubt, bravado and experimentation. Young people are very vulnerable during this period of extreme change. Their emerging voices need to be treated with the utmost respect and encouragement.

A blank piece of paper

When working with writing and young people, it is important to begin by capturing their imagination. The images conjured up by young people in response to the idea of 'poetry' tend to be of dusty old books and boredom. At Poetry Slam, we begin with an example of performance poetry by presenting a RAP (rhythm and poetry) to the workshop participants. For example:

We murdered the Alphabet one letter at a time
And we'll tell you 'bout how we committed this crime.
I assassinated A, I busted up B
And as you can C, I D-stroyed D.
I exterminated E, we fought with F,
Wee-wicky-wee-wa,
We flung it to its death.
GHI, garrotted and hung them.
JK Rowling L and M,
We were badder than Eminem.

By the time the young people have finished listening to the poem, their stock images of dusty books and boredom have been altered. RAP is a popular contemporary art form accepted by young people, and it has connotations of rebellion. It also stretches and plays with the boundaries and rules of language. This reflects adolescents' behaviour as they are exploring boundaries in their own lives; they participate in a group experience of enjoying the dexterity of language.

As George Orwell commented 'When I was sixteen, I suddenly discovered the joy of words, i.e. the sounds and associations of words'.[4]

Adolescents also tend to be captivated by their 'teachers' turning themselves into entertainers. Workshop participants appreciate that the facilitators have taken a risk in exposing themselves.

A live presentation is usually followed by a game in which ground rules are established, engendering an environment of fairness. It is also important to play a game in order to encourage a sense of fun that is associated with the creative process. Movement and laughter allow tensions in the body to release and leave individuals more willing to try something different. A workshop begins with the facilitator sharing, risk taking, giving and demonstrating even-handedness, providing a fun environment and never a direct demand for writing. As Glenn Carmichael writes in his book of poems, *The Truth is Optional*:[5]

I dare not think of the time spent
Staring at a blank piece of paper
And the blank piece of paper
Stares back
A blank stare.
(Glenn Carmichael)

My experience of presenting young people with a blank piece of paper is, indeed, a blank stare in return.

There is an exercise that was introduced to me by poet Mahendra Solanki during a talk on the Poetry Society's poetry class (a scheme introducing poets into schools). The exercise involves writing a noun on the left-hand edge of a long strip of paper, for example a name, a star, a window, a book, a poem. Class participants are asked to write a poetic (non-literal) definition (such as, book – somewhere you would find a story).

All the participants write their definitions on the long strip of paper, next to the noun. Then they tear the paper between the nouns and the definitions and pass the noun to their neighbour. The participants match up their new noun with the old definition, resulting in poetic statements, which can be put together as a poem:

A name – something to wish upon
A star – a view to another world
A window – somewhere you'd find a story
A book – a few special words to remember
A poem – you call me and I come

Immediately, the participants are introduced to the ideas proposed by Arieti: 'free-thinking' and 'being in a state of readiness for recognising similarities'.[2] Fresh connections are made and participants recognise their capacity for lateral and creative thought. This is an empowering exercise that can be used at the beginning of a workshop to give participants confidence in saying things that are not clichés. This exercise can be extended by asking participants to use their newly created line as the first line of a poem of their own.

Making a mark

It is important that young people are offered the right balance of structure and freedom in order to have the confidence to make a mark of their own. Writing creatively is not like maths or even writing an analytical English essay, where certain answers earn points. Creative writing is an opportunity to be individual. As Krishnamurti comments, this is contradictory to a lot of conventional education:

Conventional education makes independent thinking extremely difficult. Conformity leads to mediocrity. To be different from the group or to resist environment is not easy and is often risky as long as we worship success.[6]

However, it is important to note that the word 'conform' comes from the Latin 'to strengthen', *confomare*. The strong structure of a school allows young people to grow within strict boundaries laid down by the system. A school is able to contain a certain amount of healthy rebellion. Although it is definitely easier for a young person to remain unobserved by following the rules and being more like their peers, every individual I have seen expressing creativity in a positive way has been supported within the educational system. In fact, it is this combination of strength in the environment and 'new ideas' that a writer encourages that makes a truly creative partnership. All the same, it remains the case that when a writer asks an adolescent to write creatively, the adolescent is being asked to take a huge risk. Trying something new, different and imaginative is similar to the youngster trying new thinking that has not emerged from parents. This may arouse feelings of guilt in individuals and it is important that these feelings can be made manageable through reassurance. One way to provide this reassurance is for the writing facilitator to offer a writing structure on which to build independent thoughts. For example, in a workshop with students at the Youth Education Service, I introduced the group to my love poem *If I Could*:[7]

> *If I Could*
>
> If I could write a poem which
> changes key in exactly the right
> places, like your favourite songs ...
>
> If I could write a poem which
> switches from major to
> minor, tossing a pebble
> in your rib cage ...
>
> If I could write a poem which
> turns heads as it walks
> down the street ...
>
> If I could write a poem which
> smiles when you fix
> your eyes on it ...
>
> If I could write a poem which
> plays drinking games with
> you when you are lonely ...
>
> If I could ...
> I would write a poem for you.
> (Williamson)

Then I asked the students to try their own poem, starting with a structure of six lines beginning 'If' and this was one of the responses:

> If I make a poem – it's got to be right.
> If it is Christmas time – where are the presents?
> If it is snowing – there could be sun shining.
> If you are driving – maybe you are tired.
> If they are right bastards – let's forgive them.
> (Gary Gardner)

The author of this poem commented, 'It was hard to do, but it was good thinking up these things that came from my head. I started with the first part of each line and kept going back and adding the second parts when the inspiration came'.

In this way, young people are shown that there is a safe path to tread, in territory that has already been explored successfully. They may be trying something new, but they are introduced to it in such a way that they feel safe and guilt is minimised.

Discovering a unique voice

Adolescents are no strangers to story-making, as George Orwell reflects on his teenage years:

> I was carrying out a literary exercise of a quite different kind: this was the making up of a continuous 'story' about myself, a sort of diary existing only in the mind. I believe this is a common habit of children and adolescents.[4]

This is what we would call a personal narrative. It is important to remember that 'narrative' (an account of events) is very much the domain of poetry. The poetic tradition was built on great poetic narratives such as Homer's *The Iliad* and *The Odyssey*. Young narrators may never want their personal narratives to see the light of day, but they may find exposure in the form of story-making or character-making for a poem. Giving 'voice' to a personal narrative can be therapeutic, as described by Celia Hunt in the context of psychotherapy: 'Personal narratives are consciously being explored for the light they can throw on present discomforts'.[8]

The page can become a private–public interface for deeply personal feelings that may not be able to find voice elsewhere: 'For abused children, poetry offers a channel for speaking of feelings when all other channels appear closed'.[3]

When writing poetry, the poem acts as a vessel into which we can pour our feelings. The raw material can then be crafted, shared and understood on a more universal level. It is a place where young people can test and establish their voices. Finding your voice, at whatever age, is an invaluable foundation on which to build your life.

However, it is impossible for a young person simply to *arrive* at their unique voice, just as children do not transform into adults overnight. As teenagers experiment, so must fledgling writers experiment on their way to finding their voices. It is important to give young people permission to write in multiple ways: poetry is versatile and far-ranging. It is the writer's role to introduce the variety of forms a poem may take. As writer Natalie Goldberg states in her advice to writers:

> We have to accept ourselves in order to write. Now, none of us does that fully; few of us even do it halfway. Don't wait for one hundred percent acceptance

of yourself before you write, or even eighty percent acceptance. Just write. The process of writing is an activity that teaches us about acceptance.[9]

It is important to emphasise that there are no right or wrong answers with creativity, and creations can remain unfinished, or many drafts may be needed in order to get anywhere near a finished product that feels true to the writer. Krishnamurti says of the 'urge to be successful':

> The urge to be successful, which is the pursuit of reward whether in the material or the so-called spiritual sphere, the search for inward and outward security, the desire for comfort – this whole process smothers discontent, puts an end to spontaneity and breeds fear; and fear blocks the intelligent understanding of life.[6]

This is very much the essence of the writer's journey. As a writing facilitator, I constantly reinforce that what we look for in new writing is a fresh and unique voice, not a regurgitation of last week's 'big success'. Through permission to experiment comes a confidence in an unfamiliar sound – a sound that is no longer childish, but has elements of adult assurance, gained through a process of self-acceptance.

An intelligent understanding of life

I have the utmost admiration for teachers in the current educational system. Their task to deliver an ever-mutating curriculum is practically impossible, like trying to fill a bucket with a hole in it. And I am not surprised that I am often greeted by a teacher informing me about the students who will not engage with me, or who will find the task too challenging. I am sure that the teacher knows how their students behave within the academic educational system, but human intelligence has so many more facets than this system reveals on a day-to-day basis. The opportunity to think imaginatively and to engage with the existential questions that poetry manages so well is not readily available to teachers.

Working with Poetry Slam, the philosophy is to encourage young people to write for a performance in front of their peers. Slam poetry is presented orally, so emphasis is 'off' good grammar and 'on' the ability of individuals to connect with people in an audience.

Writing poetry requires thought and imagination. Performing poetry demands overcoming fear, being disciplined and having immense courage. To present a poem means employing techniques of body language, voice intonation, gestures and facial expressions: all of these are useful in the real world. Once someone begins rehearsing a poem that they have written, they are embarking on a journey of discovery that is truly character building. The idea is that everyone in a class contributes to writing a poem (often as a group) and then everyone helps in the presentation of that poem. The different strengths within a group find expression in a range of roles, so a participant can adopt one of the following: speaker, mime artist, dancer, singer, introducer, beat-box, sound effect. The results produce radically different art works, ranging from wistful nature-inspired poems to noisy RAPs. What the audience sees is not the imperfections of the individual, but the synchronicity of the group as one 'poetry organism'. What is most evident is how varied – yet equally engaging – each piece can be. One student commented:

> It has made me enjoy more types of poems. Everyone did something differ-ent. It gave me good social skills and made me more confident and happy to perform in front of an audience.
> (Liam Ring)

The result of participating in and witnessing a Poetry Slam is to observe that it is OK and even enjoyable to be different. This is an important and healing les-son against the tide of peer group pressure that sweeps through many educational establishments.

Another student commented:

> I really enjoyed watching other people's poems being performed and perform-ing our own. I noticed as we went along, people got a lot more confident and carried on even when we made mistakes. I really enjoyed today's workshop and hope I can do another one again.
> (Lydia Purcell)

And a teacher's feedback:

> There is little opportunity in the curriculum for this kind of activity and so I feel the students benefited greatly. Thanks!
> (Emily Walsh)

The opportunity for young people to explore a different side to themselves and see hidden qualities in one another opens their minds to embrace their peers through a new set of values.

Audience and applause

In 2005, I worked with Welsh National Opera and young people from various schools and colleges in the Rhondda Valley, who had been brought together for a week-long half-term workshop. The week was facilitated by a variety of profes-sionals, including composers, dramatists and singers, and I represented the writing element. The participants were self-selecting and arrived with appro-priate enthusiasm, which allowed the creative team to move their current creative experience on to new terrain. The project, entitled 'Wozzeck Songlines', aimed to respond to the opera *Wozzeck*, written in 1925 by German composer Alban Berg (1885–1935), and the result would be a 20-minute piece to be performed in the impressive foyer of the Wales Millennium Centre. It was essential that the young people did not engage solely with creative processes, but were disciplined enough to create and rehearse a finished product suitable for public performance. Performing in public is a highly exposing experience that, if managed correctly, can be amazingly rewarding for young people.

Wozzeck is a challenging opera, based on a true story, with themes that include love, betrayal, mental instability, poverty and parenthood. All of them are relevant to young people who are about to enter an adult world. It was important to give the workshop participants a non-threatening introduction to lyric writing. Rather than introduce this German opera to them immediately, I selected extracts of music by Berg, to which I wrote easily accessible lyrics in English representing the four emotions that we chose to explore: love, loyalty, control of life, and fear. The piece about fear was only two lines long:

Fear's sharp claws in me!
Fear rips, its grip I breathe.

In response to these lines, we thought of words associated with *fear* and chose one word each to say with expression. Then we took the initial sound of the word (for example, *terror* – 'te', *claustrophobia* – 'clau') and expressed it, showing the expression of the word through a physical pose. This created the jerky lines: 'Te-te-te-te/Clau-clau-clau-clau'. We proceeded by talking about how fear was presented through the body, and the group members suggested heavy breathing. This introduced the idea of spelling out F–E–A–R through heavy breathing. The words began to flow from these two ideas. We had already discussed the idea of originality and avoiding clichés, so the group members were careful to put slightly unexpected words together. We talked about the most scary sounds that we had heard and one participant said that he found children singing nursery rhymes very creepy, so we added the nursery rhyme and it was agreed that there would be a pause in the music while acapella voices sang the words to the rhyme. Below is the resulting lyric, which was set to drums and electric guitar:

Ef-Ee-Aa-Ar (heavy breathing)
Mmmmmmm (a low hum)
Mental shutdown
Beyond the limit
Self implosion
Ef-Ee-Aa-Ar
Mmmmmmm
Te-te-te-te

Clau-clau-clau-clau
Claustrophobia
Fear of small spaces
Imagination overload
Ring a ring of roses
A pocket full of posies
Atishoo! Atishoo!
We all fall down
Ef-Ee-Aa-Ar
Mmmmmmm
Like a shadow
always behind
Petrified
Foul like death
Blood pulsing through your head
Desert sand
Cold sweat in your hand
Pins and needles
Blood running cold
Shiver!

Group members commented:

> I feel this song is very powerful. It shows true feeling and emotion at the same time. It portrays fear very well.
> (Thomas Tudor Jones, Welsh speaker, aged 13)

> I feel this song is very fantastic and fearful. The style of music we are singing it with shows off the emotion of the song very well. I really enjoyed making this piece.
> (Katie Jane Davies, aged 13)

One group of girls was faced with the challenging topic of 'control of life'. They had lots of great ideas, but they could not decide what to commit to paper. There was a lot of heated discussion about who was right, although all the girls had very similar ideas. We decided to take one word that they all agreed upon, *stronger*, to write lyrics acrostically. This means writing the word vertically down the left-hand edge of the page and using each letter to begin a sentence. This formula gave a very clear structure to the exercise. Roberto Assaglioli comments on this technique in his book *The Act of Will*, which is concerned with self-actualisation: 'The act of precise formulation also helps us to curb the often restless overactivity of the mind and compels it to think in an orderly way'.[10]

The focus was immediately regained and the lyrics were written within minutes. They read as follows:

So I'm feeling stronger as the days go by
Time is on my side and I'm in control
Reality is knocking at my door
Only I can make my world go around
No one can stop me I'm stronger now
Give me power, strength to hold my head up high
Everyone has responsibilities
Regrets are nothing all I need to be is stronger

The participants commented:

> I enjoyed performing this song, as it feels it has a good vibe to it. The words make me sit up and take notice.
> (Nikki Davies)

> I felt this song describes someone with complete control of their life. All the words meant being in control.
> (Emma Edwards)

> I feel that the lyrics in this song really describe 'control of life'. The lyrics are really strong and powerful. I have enjoyed writing and singing the song.
> (Jess Nadal)

The workshop participants were able to show off their potential in a high-profile public event, backed by Welsh National Opera, and they had a real sense of ownership of the songs. It was an evening where young people truly shone and the audience was delighted to see young people performing their own songs. The young people's efforts were rewarded with excellent feedback and rapturous applause.

Conclusion

Poetry is about the life experience. It reminds us what it is to be human and how challenging that can be for all of us at times, but especially as teenagers. Poetry is about embracing life and love, and letting go of fear. The creative process parallels the foundation of a clear and solid sense of self, allowing for play, openness, free thinking, discipline, risk taking, trust, exploring boundaries, making fresh connections, experimentation, self-acceptance and realising potential.

References

1 Flint R (2004) The healing innerscape. *Lapidus* **8**: 6–8.
2 Arieti S (1976) *Creativity: the magic synthesis*. Basic Books, New York.
3 Mazza N (2003) *Poetry Therapy: theory and practice*. Brunner Routledge, Hove.
4 Orwell G (1947) *Why I Write*. Penguin, London.

5 Carmichael G (1995) *The Truth is Optional.* POTA Press, Bristol.
6 Krishnamurti J (1955) *Education and the Significance of Life.* Victor Gollancz, London.
7 Williamson C (2003) *If I Could.* In: Prausnitz M (ed.) *Velocity.* Black Spring Press, London.
8 Hunt C (2000) *Therapeutic Dimensions of Autobiography in Creative Writing.* Jessica Kingsley, London.
9 Goldberg N (1991) *Wild Mind.* Rider Books, London.
10 Assaglioli R (1990) *The Act of Will.* Crucible, London.

CHAPTER 12

The art of memory: poetry and elderly people

Graham Hartill

An aged man is but a paltry thing,
A tattered coat upon a stick, unless
Soul clap its hands and sing, and louder sing
For every tatter in its mortal dress.
(William Butler Yeats, *Sailing to Byzantium*, 1928)

Introduction

Growing old, and working with people who are already old, involves negotiation with the fundamental issues of life and death. Poetry is capable of dealing with the profundity of such issues.

For seven years I worked as a facilitator for the Ledbury Poetry Festival, working with elderly people on what came to be known as the 'Life-lines' project. My colleague, Fiona Sampson, and I would go forth into the community to take the work of the festival to a section of the public who might all too easily be excluded. We found ourselves bringing poetry back into the wider public arena: poetry written by people we had met and talked to, and poetry written down by us after conversations and reminiscence sessions. In this chapter I want to discuss our methods and introduce some ideas arising from them, and I hope its worth and the need to develop this kind of work wherever possible are conveyed to the reader.

Working with elderly people involves particular challenges: there may be practical difficulties arising from physical problems, such as loss or impairment of sight, hearing and mobility, as well as a massive variety of illnesses. Significantly for us, as poets, they may also have cognitive losses and, although it may be glib to claim that illness brings power to poetry, memory loss most certainly can do this. I will dwell on this aspect of our work for two reasons. First, it has consequences for the way we produce and regard poetry that is generated within the verbal arts in healthcare, therapy and personal development. Second, because cognitive losses are a growing problem and, of course, an extremely distressing one, for carers, relatives and loved ones as well as 'sufferers'.

I have worked with elderly people in a wide variety of settings: clubs, drop-in centres, Alzheimer's groups, residential settings, people's houses, stroke units and hospital wards. Other practitioners have worked in hospices. As well as the interests and needs of the participants, each situation determines the kind of work we do there. We can work with groups and individuals and, ideally, with both. We can have 'presentation' sessions, by which I mean giving a reading or talk and inviting responses and conversation, or we can have creative sessions, where poetry may be generated through a variety of means. However, the best situations occur when the feeling and the attention within the room are such that the whole occasion feels like a poetic experience. I do not mean this in a pretentious way; I am speaking of a situation that feels comfortable and creative, in which a 'higher' register of discussion, of listening and speaking takes place, where people feel that their input is listened to and appreciated, and where they are free to talk about more personal or important, more profound, things.

So what do we, as facilitators and participants, hope to get out of these experiences? The answers are many and varied. One is simply having a good time: to get together with others in an enjoyable and positive way that enhances and entertains us. Participants should feel that they can join in as well as they are able, that they are not excluded through carelessness or lack of consideration. A second answer is creative pleasure: that we have achieved, either alone or in collaboration with others, a meaningful form of self-expression. There will surely be an enhanced sense of self-worth as a result of this. Thirdly, we may increase our understanding and involvement in life and death.

Going about it

Jenny is 102. She is bright of mind but cannot get about on her own. She lives in a residential home and twice a week goes to the day-centre where she sits with 20 other elderly people. Activities take place there and meals are provided. Jenny can always be found at the table next to the window; an individual's seat is always sacrosanct.

I enter the room and have a cup of tea and a chat with the staff. I am announced, usually in an embarrassing way, as 'the poet' or '... who has come to read some poetry to us today!'. Actually that is not what I am going to do but I am prepared and offer a rendition of one or two favourites, such as Wordsworth's *Daffodils* (written in 1815 and indexed as 'I wandered lonely as a cloud' because it has no title), which are guaranteed to go down well. I tell everyone what I am there to do and who I represent: the Poetry Festival and what goes on there. Usually, no one in the room would ever consider actually going to a festival event; some have never even heard of it! I aim to be friendly and completely non-threatening, and say that I am going to be popping in from time to time and I am interested in hearing any stories or life events that anyone wants to tell me about. I explain that I am just going to mingle, drink some tea and maybe even stay for lunch. When hymns are sung on special occasions, I sing them, too; when raffles are held, I buy a ticket. People start to talk to me as I get to know them. I write things down, perhaps tape-record them, with permission of course. And stories happen.

I go and sit by Jenny. She does not hear very well so I hope that her favourite worker, Mandy, is there to help me out. I ask her, 'How long have you lived in Ledbury, Jenny?' and we are away. It is important not to tire her: patience is a most important tool. But, suddenly, something startling is said, 'Talking of stepfathers, my stepfather was my boyfriend'.

What? What have we stumbled on here? Is this going to be sensational and acutely private? No, as it turns out, but it is a little story full of history, personal and social, a snapshot of family life and its timeless complexity. In other words, a poem may be born from it.

Listening

I am being subjective here. I am a poet; I want to admit to that, and I am careful not to present myself as a therapist, a social worker, a care worker or a passive entity. I am there with an agenda. What I do is collaborate. And what the participants are invited to do is collaborate with me, and each other, on a poetic enterprise. So what do I listen out for? How do I deal with what I hear, and what do we make together?

I listen for good stories: tales that speak to me and others in this room and beyond, tales of real life. I listen for speech: the music of language, the interesting phrase, the music of ordinary speech. I listen for imagery: the telling detail, the striking picture, the bright moment of memory. I jot down or record what I hear. I show my respect for those I meet by trying to give them my full attention, by bearing witness to what they have to say and the words they use.

The process of writing down is commonly known as 'scribing'.

Transcribing

Then there is the business of *doing* something with these words. Anyone who has ever transcribed a passage of spoken words from tape to page will know the amount of work involved in this, and the tediousness of attending to every detail. There is no objective, 'true' transcription: words are uttered in a room, with others around; with tea or pills intervening; digressions, distractions and all the business of life. The written word is produced at a desk, usually via a machine, in a certain font, on a piece of paper, and it is meant to be read. It is a different animal. Something has been *trans*-scribed, that is, has been brought from one condition to another, the way a translated poem both *is* and *is not* the original.

The poetic *process* is not the same as when we write our own poems at home; it has a different kind of complexity. Relationship and collaboration, and the honour we pay to those processes, are crucial to our enterprise. We have to stand up and be counted as poets because the way we go about this business and the outcomes of it will be deeply influenced by our own techniques, our interests and expectations. But, here, poetry is not just defined as a finished piece but as *a series of different, related processes and presentations.* Because of this I want to claim that this kind of work reclaims some notions of poetry that have been lost in a culture where the individual's orderly, 'completed' and decorous work is the dominant paradigm.

This is a poem from *Life-lines*,[1] which was transcribed in the way I have described:

> My stepfather was my boyfriend.
> He was 19, I was 16,
> and I went with him.
>
> When Father died
> (he was never the same since the war)
> he proposed to Mother.
> Then she died.
> She was 49.
>
> Then one day he came in the shop
> and said right,
> I'm going to marry you!
> I said he blooming well wasn't!
>
> He's over Hereford way.
> I told them not to tell him
> that Jenny was still alive.
> (Jenny, '102')

Poetic process

To recapitulate, the essential stages of this kind of work, as I have come to understand them, are:

- listening
- scribing
- transcribing
- presenting back to participants for their approval, qualification, addition, modification and permission to use in readings or publication (may be repeated several times)
- readings and/or publication.

In group situations, we might read a poem and receive a lot of input, primarily about its content, from the group. I suggest that everything that happens when you or participants present a poem *is* the poem. Publication is only one aspect of it: not so much the primary or final outcome, as it is commonly regarded in literary terms, but a moment in the life of a poem. A poem is still continuing, now as you read it; in fact, the poetic *process* will go on indefinitely.

Here is a second scenario: I walk into a care home and I am introduced to Maggie – having been told that she is a bit 'confused'. In fact, it quickly becomes apparent that Maggie's dementia is quite advanced. But she is self-controlled and more than willing to talk. She does not mind, or care, about the tape-recorder, so I switch it on. For the next half-hour she talks in an authentic 'stream of consciousness' in which places and people are jumbled up in a seeming welter of history and fantasy. I want to present a longish sample from the transcription poem I produced from this encounter,[1] as it raises a lot of pertinent questions and problems concerning both aesthetics and ethics.

> Solomon's Tump I was born,
>   in 1906 I know.
> I was 92 just after Christmas.
> I've been down here a few years,
> lived through two world wars,
> I don't want to see another.
>
> I lived in Solomon's Tump.
> We used to walk in those days to Ebbw Vale,
>   over the mountain.
> We never noticed it,
> we preferred to walk.
>
> I was walking home one night from work,
> I knew that there was someone following me.
> I turned round and all I could see was something white,
>   that's why I ran.
>
> And then a little man come
> and I screamed –
> he said no–no–no
>   it's all right.
> It was a spy.
>
> We were all in the pits.
> I lived there from a very young age,
> I was cheeky, I was the nosy one.
> There's always a nosy child I reckon.
>
> I heard the one voice,
>   just one word I heard.

I asked mam, I said it,
    am I clever?

Damn what did you say?
Then he said,
    what did you do that for?
You shouldn't have said that.

Well, what was it then?

I bought a little gun,
a little Amchester-Brewster it was.
He said what have you got that for?
I said, I'll shoot *you* if you don't shut up, I said to my brother.

It was dangerous for him.
Four sisters
and two brothers.
It was happy days then although they were dangerous,
    you pulled the one with the other.

I'm 90-odd, I don't know.
I don't want a telegram from her.

Peggy's Pit they called the pit my dad used to work in.
My dad would go down in Tredegar
and he'd come out at the top of my garden,
nearly 3 mile.

That was when I was living on top up there,
    on Solomon's Tump.
We had lovely gardens –
blackcurrants, redcurrants, gooseberries, raspberries.

My father worked in Peggy's Pit.
I was down the pit at first
then I was on top of the pit.
I was cutting coal,
– cutting, bagging, selling.
A really hard life.
We didn't mind, it was hard work,
dangerous work.
We loved our work and that was it.
(Maggie, excerpt from *Solomon's Tump*)

I have quoted this poem at length because it raises important issues about what we may regard as poetry in this context. It does not follow a conventional struc-ture, it is not chronological or even consistent in its point of view; in fact, it is 'all over the place'. But only in a sense. These words were all spoken by one individual: nothing has been added to them; they tell various stories simultaneously and may be seen as truer to life, or to thought, than any simple reduction to convenient pattern or meaning. The poetry here lies in the immediacy of the images and the rhythms, and the intrigue they create in our minds. It demands that we, like the poet John Keats, be open to 'negative capability', which he defined as our being 'capable of being in uncertainties, mysteries, doubts, without any irritable reaching after fact and reason'. People who have dementia are often beyond fact and reason, but, contrary to what we might expect, within such difficult conditions the stuff of poetry may be found. *Solomon's Tump* is, in my view, every bit as true to this particular life as any more ordinary life; it is not so much a transcription of the mental derangements of dementia as an honest tribute to the wonders of language when freed from the shackles of predictability.

Whose poetry?

It is important to me that facilitators working with older people are aware of their role. It is surely disingenuous to deny that we are taking part at the most fundamental level in the making of the poetry. As soon as we walk in the room we have an effect: we arrive with an agenda. As soon as we put pen to paper we are *doing* poetry, the poetry is ours as well as theirs. But, for me, the key is collaboration; this is poetry made between people, made from conversation and the play of words. Our skill is in making a situation participatory for all concerned and in seeking a truth that is based on respect for both the person and the language we all are part of.

During a project at Leeds General Infirmary in the autumn of 2004, freelance practitioner Sue Wood felt the need to write her own poems as well as transcription poems from her meetings there. As she says, you are a poet all the time, even when you are only getting a cup of water! This is not a facetious comment; as the poet Rose Flint also stresses, what you bring to the encounter is, first and foremost, your enthusiasm for, and your commitment to, poetry.[2] This is your offering to your clients. Once accepted, in whatever form, it belongs to everyone involved, despite the peculiarities and difficulties of any particular situation.

Here, Sue Wood writes about the first hurdle she encountered, a fundamental one:

> I was thrown by the feeling that I should be encouraging patients to keep to our agreed 'theme' of holidays and felt it was inconsiderate to talk too firmly or keep coming back to *my* task (after all, the exercise is for the patients, not me). The first patient, Grace, was impossible to lead into any story other than her own account of experiences. I was so concerned about the visit not working to theme that I missed what was lively and colourful amongst her many

repetitions. I feel sorry for this. I left feeling that all I had done was to listen. It was a peculiarly alienating experience in which I shut down. Grace is very deaf. On reflection I realise her mode of continuous monologue is a way of connecting to the world that she hears poorly. She asked if she was boring us and I felt guilty. My three other visits restored my confidence. I listened better, attended to the rhythms of speech and repetition so, as I wrote I was trying to capture something of the person in their voice.[3]

Thus, Sue Wood came to work successfully with another aspect of 'negative capability', producing some fine work as a result:

For Mary, Ward 26

You sit, frail as a grass stem
bent against yourself.
Leaning sideways, you look at tomorrow
which stands behind you,
a grey shape with no name.

I ask you to name the shape.
You give it words.
I hear your words, catch them
for a moment in the air.

I touch your arm.
You look away from the postcard
of striped deck chairs facing
an empty blue sea that I give to you.

'I don't know,' you say.
(Sue Wood)

Whose therapy?

No one can get any younger, and no one recovers from Alzheimer's disease, so what do we mean by therapy here? A simple definition may be 'making better'. But who better? What better?

I started by making a rather big statement: 'Growing old, and working with people who are already old, involves negotiation with the fundamental issues of life and death. Poetry is capable of dealing with the profundity of such issues'. It is obvious that we all must die, but what do I mean by 'negotiation'? Death holds all the cards, it is true, but death defines our lives, and while we are still alive we can use the practice of art to understand our lives and the part death will play in it. We may die as individuals but those we love, or know, live on and carry us with them; they carry stories about us with them: life-stories, life-lines.

Thus, our lives, like words, are never owned by us. Life, it seems to me, is a continual state of 'coming to terms' (quite literally, 'finding the words') with which to tell ourselves, and others, about our lives.

Poetry means 'to shape, to make', and *healing* means to 'make whole'; the etymological likeness of these words is striking. And *therapeutic* means 'pertaining to the healing art', and thus the equation is completed. Surely, in the broadest terms, it is client, practitioner and, significantly, family and friends who are made more whole by our work, done well.

Conclusion

I have only had time in this chapter to make a few broad claims for the purpose of poetry work with elderly people, and to stress the importance of the relationship between client, poet and reader. It is a field still in its infancy and its possibilities for growth are endless.

One thing is certain: there is no shortage of demand. The elderly population is expanding steadily, resources are stretched and more and more elderly people live in jeopardy, not just of forgetfulness but of being forgotten. I do not just mean in the literal sense of not being properly cared for, but in a cultural sense; their self-expression in words, what Yeats called 'Soul', descending into oblivion. In a culture of transient gratification, young and old are both the worse for that.

References

1   Hartill G (2003) *Life-lines: transcription poems from the Ledbury Poetry Festival.* Ledbury Poetry Festival.
2   Flint R (2004) Fragile space: therapeutic relationship and the word. In: Sampson F (ed.) *Creative Writing and Social Care.* Jessica Kingsley, London.
3   Wood S (2004) *Acute Elderly: a short writing project for TONIC at Leeds General Infirmary, September–October 2004.* Project diary.

CHAPTER 13

Poetry in counselling training

Education is not the filling of a pail, but the lighting of a fire.
(William Butler Yeats)

Introduction

A significant part of counselling and psychotherapy training is what is known as personal development or self-development. It is the part that addresses the Ancient Greek injunction, 'know thyself', which puts a high value on self-awareness. The reason behind this is that counsellors and therapists are involved in interpersonal encounters with their clients: they need to be attuned to what their clients are saying; they need to know when clients are 'sparking off' difficult feelings in them; they need to be aware of when they feel uneasy, for instance if clients become angry or manipulative, and how they respond to this. They should be aware of how they react when a client expresses political views that are directly at odds with their own. They need to know the sort of client who evokes a sense of identification or protectiveness, or boredom.

Trainees also need to have explored at first hand painful conflicts they are still carrying around, for instance unresolved losses or a need for approval or gratitude from their clients. Most awarding bodies follow the British Assocation for Counselling and Psychotherapy (BACP) (www.bacp.co.uk) requirement that a quarter of a counselling course consists of activities connected with personal development.[1]

Course tutors address these needs through various channels but the main ones are:

- exercises promoting self-awareness and self-understanding
- personal development groups
- trainees undergo individual therapy
- journal writing
- input during the course on creative themes, such as art, music or poetry.

The last two are those focused on in this chapter, but first it is worth considering briefly where the strengths and weaknesses of personal development groups and individual therapy lie.

Personal development groups

The great value of personal development groups, when they work well, is that they can be a living demonstration of how individuals carry defences, how they project feelings and issues onto other people and others do the same to them. They offer a chance, if people are able to be honest, for real change in self-perception and the perception of others to take place. Often, a great feeling of closeness and intimacy develops through the shared experience.

At worst, personal development groups can be quite damaging for some individuals, especially if there is an element of hostility that is never resolved or if maladaptive roles are reinforced (for instance, if a member of the group insists on being a 'mother figure', so that she does not ever have to make herself vulnerable, and the group reinforces that role). Sometimes they are simply ineffective as they never get past the social chit-chat phase and some members end up feeling frustrated and experience the group as a waste of time.

Individual therapy

Many counselling courses now insist on trainees having their own therapy, and all psychotherapy courses make it a basic requirement. Apart from the opportunity it offers for self-exploration, undergoing therapy gives trainees the experience of being clients, and how it feels to make a relationship with a therapist. The individual works through concerns such as apprehension, ambivalence, strong positive and negative feelings towards the therapist. If fortunate, trainees learn things that are valuable when they become counsellors. Being on a counselling or psychotherapy course often stirs up issues where it is essential to get some individual support and gain insight.

Because the therapy takes place away from the college, it is harder for tutors to assess its effectiveness. Sometimes trainees are just 'going through the motions' to satisfy the requirements of the course, sometimes they go to a therapist who does not have a lot to offer and they become quite disillusioned.

Journal writing

Journal writing started as a therapeutic tool in working with clients and was only later adapted for use on counselling courses. Kate Thompson describes it as 'a means of establishing relationships with the self and with others'.[2] In therapy it has the advantage of always being available to the individual as a resource; journals can be written immediately or soon after thoughts, feelings or conflicts arise, and they are a record so that individuals can see recurring themes or ways in which they have changed or developed.

These benefits are the same ones that arise in counselling training. Most trainees are enthusiastic about the positive part their journal has played in their ability to express difficult and complex emotions about the course, about their personal lives and especially about how the past is affecting their present. Daniels and Feltham (2004) asked students to identify the advantages of journal writing as a means of personal development, and they report, 'Key words used included: time/space, reflection, a means of clarifying thinking, expressing and identifying feelings, confidential, honest, freedom of expression'.[3]

One trainee who was coming to the end of a course in which there had been a number of difficulties wrote in her journal:

This week I write for the last time in my journal:

We are close to an ending
But without ending
The beginning felt wrong
But appeared not to be wrong;
Different tutors, a demanding group
I have learned so much

There was a lot of power
Positive power, negative power
Useless power and useful power
How closely is trust, safety, linked to power.
I have learned so much

End of a journal, end of two years
An ending, not just ending
An ending that contains beginning
The beginning of the next process
The cycle that does not contain an ending
I have learned so much.

Having taught on courses where the tutor reads the trainee's journal, I always find it quite staggering how much of trainees I did not know until that point, even though I thought I knew them. It reminds me of the proverbial iceberg with so much going on beneath the surface. Sharing a journal with a tutor demands a very high level of trust, especially in the rare cases where a trainee disagrees with a tutor or a college, but it does make possible a much closer working alliance. It is also the area of the written part of the course in which trainees can be much freer in their expression and legitimately go off on tangents. All the benefits of creative expression that are explored elsewhere in this book apply when keeping a journal: managing your thoughts, having a dialogue with yourself and being flexible in your means of self-expression.

It is very common for trainees to write poetry in their journals, or to include a poem that means a great deal to them. This, in turn, encourages them to help clients see the therapeutic benefit of self-expression.

Input on training of creative topics

The degree to which counselling and psychotherapy courses include creative approaches varies enormously. There is a danger that trainees, having done one workshop on, say, sculpting or art therapy, think that they are trained in the subject. However, the whole ethos of a psychotherapy or counselling training course is to encourage trainees to reflect on where they are professionally: what their strengths and limitations are, and what they still need to know and experience. This should act as a safeguard against overconfidence. With this proviso, demonstrating and exploring other ways of working with troubled or questioning individuals is very productive.

An important thing for trainees to realise is that, just as there are a wide variety of counselling and psychotherapy models, so there are many therapeutic ways of working with people. The way the body moves, heightened states of awareness, drama, colour, textures, music, literature and spiritual awareness are all part of our physical and emotional way of being. Introducing some of these areas makes trainees aware that they, too, can benefit from exploring what increases their sense of well-being. Within the BACP ethical framework one of the values is listed as, 'Appreciating the variety of human experience and culture' and under its section on ethical principles it states, 'The principle of self-respect encourages active engagement in life-enhancing activities and relationships that are independent of relationships in counselling or psychotherapy'.[1] The solitary nature of counselling makes it all too easy for counsellors to become stale or unadventurous.

Professional development

Both the BACP and the United Kingdom Council for Psychotherapy (UKCP) (www.psychotherapy.org.uk) require accredited practitioners to show evidence of ongoing professional development in order to continue to be accredited. It is now recognised that counsellors tend to become more eclectic as they become more experienced. Roth and Fonagy (1996), who showed that the 'therapeutic alliance' was the greatest factor in effective therapy, not technique, also found that 'differences between theoretical models become less and less as practitioners become more experienced'.[4] This suggests that as practitioners become more confident they are prepared to try out new ideas and new techniques. Hollanders (1997) found that the primary reason for this extension of technique was in response to the need of the client.[5] In other words, it seems that the approaches therapists used did not always work and that therapists extended their range of interventions. An example of this might be a therapist who finds her conventional way of working with someone with an eating disorder ineffectual, and who then trains in a technique of using 'body imaging'.

Poetry and other literature in counselling training

With this idea in mind – that counsellors and psychotherapists become more eclectic and more adventurous with experience – when is the right time to introduce literature and other creative arts into counselling training? My feeling is that they belong towards the latter part of a training course, once trainees have a good grounding in theory, skills development, and professional and ethical issues. Creative arts can also play a large part in post-qualification training. However, tutors, like counsellors, have their own individual styles, ethos and interests. Just as some tutors and counsellors show a flair for colour and textures in their dress, or pictures they hang on the wall, so some tutors will share their enthusiasm for art, literature or music and include it in their teaching. Because literature is very central to my life, I tend to refer to novels, poems or biographies, to ask students what they enjoy reading and to encourage discussion of books and television programmes.

To think as broadly as possible, to see connections between psychological ideas and their expression in literature, to open ourselves up to experience, is all part of counselling training. One of the best descriptions of an oedipal conflict comes in the autobiography, *And When Did You Last See Your Father?* by Blake Morrison.[6] The author, constricted by an overinvolved father, who nevertheless constantly competes with his son, describes a particularly dire family skiing holiday. He meets an attractive young girl his own age. One day his father stays behind from the skiing, pleading a strained back. On their return that evening Morrison describes the scene:

> Back in the room, at dusk, my father and Rachel are sitting on the balcony: they have drinks in their hands and are smoking and, with the mountains and ice-blue skies beyond, look like a Martini advertisement. I pour myself a whisky. I look at the bed – unrumpled, but they'd have had time to straighten it, so who can tell. I feel a sudden disgust – not just with him, for stealing Rachel before I could even get hold of her, but with her, for her sophistication and cosmopolitanism and orphan's wide-eyed fascination with an older man. As soon as I can, I flounce off.[6]

These well-written descriptions are often as good or better illustrations of psychological phenomena than client material in counselling books. In my view, one of the reasons that Irvin Yalom is so popular with counsellor trainees is that he is such an excellent writer. He manages to convey the dynamic interaction between a client and therapist and bring alive case material and human dilemmas.

Poetry workshops

As stated, I think specific inputs on music, drama or literature are best introduced towards the end of counselling or psychotherapy training. Apart from anything else, there is so much else to fit into the training programme. When running such workshops on diploma or post-qualification courses, I usually give the aims of the course as:

- increasing self-awareness
- exploring other ways of communicating
- exploring possible ways of working with clients
- focusing on metaphor and other imagery.

I usually start by asking trainees how they feel about poetry and what they feel it can achieve in ways of communication that other 'word forms' cannot. The group often falls into two camps: those people who are already enthusiastic about poetry, who loved doing it at school and have carried on reading it, and those who look studiously at the carpet, terrified they are going to be asked to recite something! I try at an early stage to make the point that, in this context, we are looking at poems as a means of relating to ourselves, our thoughts and feelings, and not as an academic exercise. I also say that no one will be asked to read out anything aloud if they do not wish to. Having said that, I have always found there are several people willing to read poems, and one aspect that usually amazes workshop participants is the passion, understanding and skill that are available within the group.

I have found that it is best to choose poems that are immediately accessible and to present a mixture of styles and content. For example, I have found that poems by Elizabeth Jennings, Wendy Cope, Robert Frost and Dylan Thomas are a good starting point. It is a good idea to have a mixture of tones: sad, humorous, energetic and reflective. At this stage the aim is simply to engage people and to see how, and if, the poems work on them. It is also effective if people both read the poems to themselves and then hear them read out loud. The sort of questions I would get people to ask themselves are:

- What appeals to me about this poem?
- Is there a phrase or image that really hit home?
- Does the mood of the poem resonate with me?
- Does the poem remind me of how I feel now or how I used to feel?
- Do the ideas of the poem resonate with me?
- Is there anything in the poem that makes me see something in a new light?

All these questions can, like a journal, reveal new, stimulating and previously unexplored aspects of trainees' development.

Another effective step is to get people to continue the discussion in pairs or threes, and to allow the conversation to develop in whatever direction it goes. Lines such as Edward Thomas', 'The Past is a strange land, most strange./Wind blows not there, nor does rain fall:', or Emily Dickinson's, 'Hope is the thing with feathers/That perches in the soul', or Wendy Cope's, 'Bloody men are like bloody buses', or Elizabeth Bishop's, 'The art of losing isn't hard to master', are all ones that can set up a rapport or tension in the listener and offer a great deal on which to focus.

Points that often emerge when people get back together and share their ideas are:

- how one image can set off a series of images
- how two people can react in a very similar or very different way to the same poem
- the memories that are provoked by an image or sound
- the overall stimulation of imaginative response
- recognition of how valuable (and how neglected) the creative part of life is
- the poem reminds them of a friend, family member or client.

There are many different ways a poetry workshop can then develop, but in making links to counselling and therapy, there are several relevant avenues.

Extending the idea of metaphor in therapeutic work

This means being attuned to the words clients use and encouraging them to stay with the metaphor and expand on them if it seems useful. Examples might include a client who talks about 'running on empty' or who has 'a mountain to climb'.

Using poetry or creative writing as part of therapy

If trainees experience for themselves how literature can enhance their awareness, express things that are otherwise hard to put into words, be a resource outside the therapeutic time, they are likely to value that way of working with their clients.

Writing as a way of self-expression

I commented in Chapter 1 that poetry is unique because reading it so often leads to writing poetry. Most people who find reading a novel an uplifting or engaging process would feel daunted at trying to write one. But people reading fine, well-crafted poetry seem to be inspired rather than put off writing it. It is certainly because a poem can be quite short, but I think it is also that the huge variety of styles and tones found in poetry make people feel they could 'have a go'.

When a workshop evolves into a creative writing workshop the facilitator needs to be aware that people are bringing to it very personal aspects of themselves, not just in content, but in whether their work will be criticised or 'good enough'.

When I have run such workshops as part of a residential course on an ongoing diploma course, I have usually found that trainees bring work in over subsequent weeks and want to share it with the group.

Pitfalls

It is important to keep the aims of the workshop in mind. Problems can arise when trainees who may have a very good grounding in literature shift the ground so that the discussion becomes more about style, syntax, a history of the Romantic movement or a biography of the poet's life. Things become too erudite and those people who have not studied literature soon feel they have no contribution to make. The focus needs to be brought back to the personal effect the poem has. Just as clients can intellectualise and thereby avoid experiencing emotions, so discussions about poetry can become academic. Many years ago Kadushin (1968) wrote an article in a social work journal called 'Games people play in supervision' one of which was called, 'If you knew Dostoievsky like I know Dostoievsky'.[7] The point made was that the trainee used her superior academic knowledge as a smokescreen for her lack of emotional confidence.

The other problem I have encountered is that a workshop becomes almost 'too successful' and that for a while the whole course turns into a creative writing class. Week after week students bring in their poems or other creative writing. It is very therapeutic for the individuals, but each piece of work takes up quite a lot of time to respond to and not all trainees want to engage in this process. It is probably better for those students who are motivated to find a creative writing course to attend as well.

Conclusion

Understandably, counselling and psychotherapy training is focused on developing skills, introducing a psychological framework and examining professional and ethical issues. However, it is important that at trainee and post-qualification level counsellors and psychotherapists are given an opportunity to value the creative part of themselves and their work. It is also helpful for them to have some exposure to how they might develop this in their work and give their clients similar opportunities.

References

1   British Association for Counselling and Psychotherapy *Ethical Framework for Good Practice in Counselling and Psychotherapy*. BACP, Rugby.
2   Thompson K (2004) Journal writing as a therapeutic tool. In: Bolton G, Howlett S, Lago C and Wright JK (eds) *Writing Cures: an introductory handbook of writing in counselling and therapy*. Brunner Routledge, Hove.
3   Daniels J and Feltham C (2004) Reflective and therapeutic writing in counsellor training. In: Bolton G, Howlett S, Lago C and Wright JK (eds) *Writing Cures: an introductory handbook of writing in counselling and therapy*. Brunner Routledge, Hove.
4   Roth A and Fonagy P (1996) *What Works for Whom? A critical review of psychotherapy research*. Guildford Press, New York and London.
5   Hollanders H (1997) Unpublished PhD thesis. University of Keele.
6   Morrison B (1993) *And When Did You Last See Your Father?* Granta Books, London.
7   Kadushin A (1968) Games people play in supervision. *Social Work* **13**: 23–32.

To conclude

Part 2 of the book has explored the power of expressive language and how individuals gain from attempting to put their thoughts and feelings into an imaginative format. There is a completion to the therapeutic process – accepting and embracing these words as 'part of you'.

As They Are

And what if my words,
my fledgling poems,
were children, were toddlers
trying first steps,
tumbling, skinning knees,
squealing with glee,
splashing mud,
making a mess,
discovering themselves?

Would I hold them
at arm's distance,
disown them, hide them,
say what I imagine
others will think –
that, after all, they
really aren't very good?

And could that be
a way of protecting them –
shielding, holding back?
I know the mockery
odd children can face.

Instead, could I let
them ramble along weedy
paths only they know?
Lean close to hear

them whisper secrets,
learn what they
need from me?
Could I love them
as they are,
give them room
to grow, a chance
to shine?
(Barbara McEnerney)

Further reading

Below are some suggestions for further reading. Each area has a vast amount of literature: this is inevitably just a signpost.

Poetry anthologies

Astley N (2002) *Staying Alive: real poems for unreal times*. Bloodaxe Books, Newcastle upon Tyne.
Astley N (2004) *Being Alive: sequel to Staying Alive*. Bloodaxe Books, Newcastle upon Tyne.
Heaney S and Hughes T (1982) *The Rattle Bag*. Faber & Faber, London.
Motion A (2001) *Here to Eternity: an anthology of poetry*. Faber & Faber, London.
Padel R (2002) *52 Ways of Looking at a Poem*. Chatto, London.
(Bloodaxe collections are particularly strong on modern poetry.)

Psychotherapy and counselling

The entire collection of Sigmund Freud's writings (24 volumes), edited by James Strachey and known as the 'Standard Edition', is published by the Hogarth Press and Vintage.

The collected works (20 volumes) of C G Jung, edited by Herbert Read, Michael Fordham and Gerhard Adler, are published by Routledge.

For a good, clear introduction see the Oxford University Press series 'A very short introduction'. The one on Freud is by Anthony Storr, that on Jung is by Anthony Stevens.

For an overview of psychotherapy and counselling theories and approaches, see *Who Can I Talk To?* by Judy Cooper and Jenny Lewis (Hodder and Stoughton) and *An Introduction to Counselling* by John McLeod (Open University Press).

For more detailed (though very accessible) expositions of particular theories and protagonists see the Sage Publications 'Counselling in action' series, in particular *Psychodynamic Counselling in Action* by Michael Jacobs, *Person Centred Counselling in Action* by D Mearns and B Thorne, *Gestalt Counselling in Action* by Petruska Clarkson, *Cognitive Behavioural Counselling in Action* by P Trower, A Casey and W Dryden, *Transactional Analysis Counselling in Action* by Ian Stewart and *Psychosynthesis Counselling in Action* by Diana Whitmore.

See also:
Bowlby J (1979) *The Making and Breaking of Affectional Bonds*. Routledge, London.
Brown D and Pedder J (1979) *Introduction to Psychotherapy*. Routledge, London.
Gomez L (1997) *An Introduction to Object Relations*. Free Association Books, London.
Rogers C (1967) *On Becoming a Person*. Constable, London.
Samuels A, Shorter B and Plaut F (1986) *A Critical Dictionary of Jungian Analysis*. Routledge, London.
Waddell M (1998) *Inside Lives: psychoanalysis and the growth of the personality*. Karnac Books, London.
West W (2004) *Spiritual Issues in Therapy*. Palgrave Macmillan, Basingstoke.
Yalom I (2002) *The Gift of Therapy*. Piatkus Books, London.

Therapy and literature

Canham H and Satyamurti C (eds) (2003) *Acquainted with the Night: psychoanalysis and the poetic imagination*. Karnac Books, London.
Cox M and Theilgaard A (1997) *Mutative Metaphors in Psychotherapy*. Jessica Kingsley, London.
Herbert WN and Hollis M (eds) (2000) *Strong Words: modern poets on modern poetry*. Bloodaxe Books, Newcastle upon Tyne.

Creative writing and personal development

Bolton G, Howlett S, Lago C and Wright JK (eds) (2004) *Writing Cures: an introductory handbook of writing in counselling and therapy*. Brunner Routledge, Hove.
Bolton G, Field V and Thompson K (eds) (2006) *Writing Works*. Jessica Kingsley Publications.
Bolton G (2011) *Write Yourself*. Jessica Kingsley Publications.
Burns L (2009) *Literature and Therapy*. Karnac Books, London.
Chavis G (2011) *Poetry and Story Therapy*. Jessica Kingsley Publishers, London.
Goldberg N (1986) *Writing Down the Bones*. Shambhala.
Hunt C and Sampson F (eds) (1998) *The Self on the Page: theory and practice of creative writing and personal development*. Jessica Kingsley, London.
Kaye C and Blee T (1997) *The Arts in Healthcare: a palette of possibilities*. Jessica Kingsley, London.
Kitwood T (2000) *Dementia Reconsidered: the person comes first*. Open University Press, Buckingham.
Mazza N (2003) *Poetry Therapy: theory and practice*. Brunner Routledge, Hove.
Phillips D, Linington L and Penman D (1999) *Writing Well: creative writing and mental health*. Jessica Kingsley, London.
Sampson F (1999) *The Healing Word: a practical guide to poetry and personal development activities*. The Poetry Society, London.
Sampson F (ed.) (2004) *Creative Writing in Health and Social Care*. Jessica Kingsley, London.

Useful websites

- American Psychotherapy Association www.americanpsychotherapy.com
- British Association of Counselling and Psychotherapy (www.bacp.co.uk)
- Canadian Counselling and Psychotherapy Association www.ccpa-accp.ca
- International Academy for Poetry Therapy www.iapoetry.org
- Literary Arts in Personal Development (www.lapidus.org.uk)
- National Association for Poetry Therapy (USA) (www.poetrytherapy.org)
- National Association of Writers in Education (www.nawe.co.uk)
- National Network for Arts in Health (www.nnah.org.uk)
- Psychotherapy Networker www.psychotherapynetworker.org
- Survivors Poetry www.survivorspoetry.org
- The Institute for Poetic Medicine (www.poeticmedicine.com)
- The Poetry Society (www.poetrysociety.org.uk)
- United Kingdom Council for Psychotherapy (www.psychotherapy.org.uk)

Index

A Child's Garden of Verses (Stevenson) 79
A Kite for Michael and Christopher
    (Heaney) 104
A Mental Hospital Sitting Room
    (Jennings) 116
A Poison Tree (Blake) 4–5
The Act of Will (Assaglioli) 130
Adcock, F 22–3
adjustments
   in adolescence 21–3
   in middle age 32–5
adolescence 19–24
   characteristics 22
   and creative work 24
   Erikson's view 21–3
   identity vs. role confusion 21–3
   life events and difficulties 23–4
   working with poetry 121–31
After Great Pain, a formal feeling comes
    (Dickinson) 57
alcohol problems, and change 78
'All the world's a stage' (*As You Like It*
    Shakespeare) 15–16
Alvarez, A 3
And When Did You Last See Your Father?
    (Morrison) 147
anger, and bereavement 57–9
Anger (Gregory) 112–13
Angus, L and Rennie, D 89
Anthem for a Doomed Youth (Owen) 69
anxiety, and spirituality 46–8
April Rise (Lee) 39
Arieti, S 121–2, 124
Arts Council 107–8
As They Are (McEnerney) *153–4*
As You Like It (Shakespeare) 15–16
aspirations and dreams, in middle age 33
Assaglioli, R 41, 130

Astley, N 12
Atlas (Fanthorpe) 52–3
attachment 51–62
   Bowlby's views 53–4
   and loss 54–61
   and love 51–3
   and parenting 29–31
Auden, WH 54–5, 66
Auguries of Innocence (Blake) 37, 54
authenticity 7–9
   and self-awareness 7–8
authority, adolescent rebellion 22–3
autonomy
   and life scripts 76–7
   stages of life (Erikson) 18–19
awareness, and creative processes 8–9

Beattie is Three (Mitchell) 29–30
Beck, AT 81
Being Fifty (Hill) 32–3
bereavement
   ambivalent feelings 67–8
   and attachment theory 53–4
   death of young people 60–1
   and dreams 9–10
   Freud's view's 55–6
   'given' losses 54–5
   moving on 64–7
   reconnecting with life 69–71
   stages of loss 56–60
   tasks of mourning 63–4
   timely or appropriate losses 60
   and 'unfinished business' 68
Berg, A 129
Berne, E 76
Berry, W 47–8
Betjeman, J 31
Blake, W 4–5, 37, 54

Bolton, G 90
boredom and listlessness 79
boundary setting 98–9
Bowlby, J 29, 53–4
brainstorming 100
Bridges, W 27
British Association for Counselling and
    Psychotherapy (BACP) 143
Brooks, G 21–2
Browning, E Barrett 52

Calman, Sir Kenneth 107
cancer care and poetry 108–11
Carmichael, G 123
Carver, R 82–3
Catcher in the Rye (Salinger) 21, 24
cathartic experiences
    cf. poetry vs. therapy 6–7
    expressions 68
Causley, C 65
Cavafy, CP 74–5
'chain of inference' (Beck) 81
change
    following injury 114
    and goals 78–9
    life transitions 16
    and parenting 29–31
Chekov, A 97
chemotherapy 111
child abuse 126
child deaths 60–1
child rearing
    cultural influences 16
    parental anxieties 29–31
childbirth 27–8
Childhood and Society (Erikson) 18
choices 80–1
cognitive behaviour therapy 81–2
Coleridge, ST 45–6
Come, My Mother's Son (Ingonga) 19–20
community healthcare settings, and
    poetry 115–16
confidentiality 99
conformity, and adolescence 23
continuing professional
    development 146–7
counselling training *see* training and
    creative writing
Crane, S 94–5

creative processes, and poetry 8–9
creative writing 6, 90–4
    and catharsis 6–7
    deep-seated feelings 102–4
    fear of judgement 94
    feedback 102
    getting started 99
    omissions 94
    reading aloud 102
    setting up groups 97–100
    and specific groups 104–5
    and 'success' 127
    techniques 100–2, 122–6
    therapist's role 93–4
creative writing groups 97–106
    boundaries and 'rules' 98–9
    setting up 97–9
    warm-up exercises 99–100
Creativity: The Magic Synthesis
    (Arieti) 121–2
creativity
    and authenticity 8–9
    key conditions 121–2
    and play 11
    therapist perspectives 10–12
culture, and life stages 16
Cummings, EE 38–9
Cymbeline (Shakespeare) 60

Daniels, J and Feltham, C 145
Dante, A 42
The Darling Letters (Duffy) 66–7
Day Lewis, C 30–1, 94
The Dead Get By With Everything
    (Holm) 57–8, 94
death
    and acceptance 60
    'relocating the deceased' 64–7
    of young people 60–1
    see also bereavement
Dejection: an Ode (Coleridge) 45–6
dementia, and creativity 137–9
depression, and spirituality 45–6
Dickinson, E 57
Dinner with my Mother (Williams) 17–18
Divine Comedy (Dante) 42
Do Not Go Gentle into that Good Night
    (Thomas) 4
Dooley, M 100–1

drama 6
dreams 9–10
about the deceased 9–10, 65–7
Drew, E 3
drug addictions, and change 78
Duffy, CA 66–7
'dumping' techniques 110–11

Eagle (Hughes) 44
Eden Rock (Causley) 65
elderly people and poetry 133–41
    creative process 136–9
    listening and transcribing 135–6
    ownership issues 139–41
    setting up sessions 134–5
Eliot, G 35
Eliot, TS 10, 48–9
Ellis, A and Bernard, ME 82
emotional numbness 57
emotional release, through writing 103–
    4
emptiness 40
Erikson, E, on life stages 18–19, 21–2, 32
'ethical commitment' (Erikson) 30
ethical considerations, poetry in
    healthcare settings 118
evaluation
    and middle age 34
    poetry in healthcare settings 118–19
The Evening Swim (Hermione) 91
Everyone Sang (Sassoon) 70
existential anxiety 47

facilitator roles, healthcare settings 117–
    18
Fanthorpe, UA 52–3
feedback, working with adolescents 127–
    8
feedback delivery 102
feelings
    communication 3–4, 6–7
    suppressed 7
    unexpressed 4–5
Feinstein, E 31–2
Feltham, C and Dryden, W 37
Fern Hill (Thomas) 43–4
Flint, R 112, 121
For Heidi with Blue Hair (Adcock) 22–3
Four Quartets (Eliot) 48–9

'free-thinking' (Arieti) 124
freedom 121
Freud, S
    on anxiety 48
    on creativity 10–11
    on 'discovering' the unconscious 3
    on dreams 9–10
    on early stages of life 17
    and human potential 40
    on mourning and bereavement 55–6, 59
From a Railway Carriage (Stevenson) 79
Frost, R 8, 12, 80
Frozen Peas (anon) 92–3

Gardner, G 125–6
general practice, and poetry projects 115
Gestalt therapy 8
Getting Older (Feinstein) 31–2
Gilbert, P 81
Give Me Back My Rags (Popa) 58
goals and aspirations 77–9
God, and spirituality 37–9
The Going (Hardy) 68
Goldberg, N 126–7
Goodbye to All That (Graves) 69
Greene, G 7
Gregory, J 112–13, 114
grief
    communicating transformation 7
    examples of creative writing 91–3
groups, and adolescence 21–3
Gunn, T 9–10, 65–6

happiness 51
Harding, G 113–14
Hardy, T 49, 67–8
healing 141
    and dreams 9–10
health, definitions 107
healthcare and poetry
    current policy climate 107–8
    cancer care settings 108–11
    community settings 115–16
    ethical considerations 118
    evaluation 118–19
    facilitators role 117–18
    mental health settings 116–17
    patient experiences 108–17
    spinal units 111–14

Heaney, S 7, 77, 104
Her First Week (Olds) 28
Hill, S 32–3, 59
Hollanders, H 146
Holm, B 57–8, 94
Homer 126
Honeymoon Flight (Heaney) 77
hope 70–1
  and loss 60–1
Hopkins, GM 4
Hughes, T 8–9, 44
human potential 40–1
human spirit
  hope and optimism 70–1
  power to endure 69–70
  as 'vital principle' 45–6
Humanist School 42–3

I Had Meant to Write (Raine) 49
identity, in adolescence 21–3
If I Could (Williamson) 125
If I Should Cast Off this Tattered Coat
    (Crane) 94–5
The Iliad (Homer) 126
imagery
  life as a journey 74–6
  and nature 43–5
  and spirituality 40
  see also metaphor use
imagination
  creative processes 8–9
  and dreams 9–10
  see also creative writing; creativity
infertility 61
Ingonga, L 19–20
'Inner Gardens' 115–16
insight, and poetry 4–5
Ithaka (Cavafy) 74–5
IVF (Macphee) 61

Jennings, E 116
Joseph, J 34
journal writing 144–6
journey of life *see* life's journey
Joyce, J 10
Jung, CJ
  on creativity 11
  on dreams 9, 66
  on Freud 40

on happiness 51
on lifespan 32
on spirituality 40–1
on transformation 87

Keats, J 44–5, 47
Kierkegaard, SA 15
Kingfisher Project (Salisbury) 112
Klein, M 11
Krishnamurti, J 124, 127
Kubler-Ross, E 56

The Lake Isle of Innisfree (Yeats) 4, 78
language use 87–90
  love of 123
  metaphors 74–6, 87–9
  pitfalls 89–90
  and poetry 5
Lapidus (Literary Arts in Personal
    Development) 85
Late Fragment (Carver) 82–3
Lawrence, DH 30
Ledbury Poetry festival 133
Leeds General Infirmary 139–40
Leedy, JJ 24
Lee, L 39
Lee, M 115
Lewis, W 109–10
life events, difficulties in
    adolescence 23–4
life scripts, and transactional
    analysis 76–7
'Life-lines' project 133–41
life's journey 73–83
  goals and aspirations 77–9
  making choices 80–1
  and therapy 74–7
  use of cognitive behavioural
    therapy 81–2
  and visions 82–3
listening and transcribing 135–6
loss
  and acceptance 60
  ambivalent feelings 67–8
  attachment theory 53
  Freud's views 55–6
  of futures 60–1
  as a 'given' 54–5
  moving on 64–7

and reconnection 69–71
sharing 64
stages 56–60
love
and attachment 51–3
parents and children 27–31
Love After Life (Walcott) 66
Lynch, W 88

Macbeth (Shakespeare) 7, 12–13
McCullers, C 21, 24
McEnerney, B 153–4
McLoughlin, D 109, 116–17
Macphee, K 61
Maslow, a 42–3
Mazza, N 24, 94–5, 122
ME (chronic fatigue syndrome), and
poetry projects 115–16
meaning explorations, cf. poetry vs.
therapy 6
Meditations in Time of Civil War
(Yeats) 59
The Member of the Wedding
(McCullers) 21, 24
memories, following spinal injury 113–
14
mental health settings and poetry 116–
17
facilitator roles 117
metaphor use 74–6, 87–9, 149
pitfalls 89–90
see also imagery; life's journey
middle age 31–5
and therapy 31–2, 34–5
Mitchell, A 29–30
mood, and rhythm of language 5
Morrison, B 147
mortality 31–2
poetry and wider contexts 69–71
mourning
ambivalent feelings 67–8
Freud's views 55–6
moving on 64–7
stages of loss 56–60
tasks 63–4
Mourning and Melancholia (Fred) 55
Multi A (Bristol) 121
My Last Walk (Harding) 13–14

National Association for Poetry
Therapy 85
National Institute for Clinical Excellence
(NICE) 107
nature and poetry 43–5
and anxiety 46–8
and depression 45–6
Noonan, E 24
Nuffield Trust, arts and humanities
initiatives 107
numbness 56–7
'numinous' 40–1

Ode. Intimations of Immortality
(Wordsworth) 46
Ode to a Nightingale (Keats) 44–5
The Odyssey (Homer) 126
oedipal complex 17
Olds, S 28
omissions 94
opera 128–31
optimism 70–1
Orwell, G 123, 126
Owen, W 69
ownership of poetry 139–40

parental love 27–31
parenting, and attachment 29–31
Parkes, CM 56
peace 79
The Peace of Wild Things (Berry) 48
'peak experiences' 42–3
personal development groups 144
Phillips, D 117
Pied Beauty (Hopkins) 4
Plato 41
play, and creativity 11
poetry qualities 141
insights 4–5
language 5
and purpose 3–5, 6–7
spirituality 37–9, 43–5
Poetry Society 123–4
poetry in therapy 87–95
attunement to language 87–9
creating work 6, 90–4
exploring deep feelings 102–4
exploring published works 94–5
ownership issues 139–40

pitfalls 89–90
and specific groups 104–5
therapists role 93–4
use with adolescents 24, 121–31
use with anxiety conditions 48
use with depressive disorders 46
use in middle age 34–5
use in old age 133–41
see also creative writing
Poetry Therapy – Theory and Practice
(Mazza) 122
poetry workshops 148–50
pitfalls 150
poets
characteristics 12
role in life (Wolberg) 63
views on therapy 12–13
Poety Slam 121–2, 127–8
Popa, V 58
pre-conscious, and language use 5
professional development 146–7
Proust, M 73
psychological pain, and creativity 12
psychosynthesis 41
Pugh, S 70

Raine, K 49
RAP (rhythm and poetry) 122–4
reading aloud 102
The Reassurance (Gunn) 9–10, 65–6
Recovery (Lewis) 109–10
regrets 31
religion, and spirituality 37–9
'relocating the deceased' 64–7
revenge 59
rhythm 5
and RAP 122–4
The Road Not Taken (Frost) 80
Rogers, CR 7, 11–12
on human potential 43
on love 52
Romeo and Juliet (Shakespeare) 60
Roth, A and Fonagy, P 146
Rowan, J 41, 43
Rowe, D 45–6

Sailing to Byzantium (Yeats) 133
Salinger, JD 21, 24
Sassoon, S 69–70

Schneider, M 110–11
self-awareness, and authenticity 7–8
self-identity, in adolescence 21–3
Shakespeare, W
As You Like It 15–16
Cymbeline 60
Macbeth 7, 12–13
Romeo and Juliet 60
Twelfth Night 7
sharing loss 64
Shikibu, I 42
Siegelman, E 87–8, 89
Solanki, M 123–4
Solomon's Tump 137–9
Sometimes (Pugh) 70
Sonnets from the Portuguese (Browning) 52
Sons and Lovers (Lawrence) 30
spidergrams 118
spinal injuries, and use of poetry 111–14
spirituality 37–49
definitions 37–8
and nature 43–8
and poetry 37–9, 43–5
religious concepts 38
and therapy 37–8, 39–43
and time 48–9
see also human spirit
staff involvement 118
stages of life 15–16, 17–18
Erikson's views 18–19, 21–2
Freud's views 17
stages of loss 56–60
Staying Alive (Astley) 12
sterotypes, in middle age 33
Stevenson, RL 79
Storr, A 10–11
'stream of consciousness' writing
approach 10, 105
stress
and goals 78
and poetry 79
substance abuse, and change 78
success, creative writing 127
suicidal ideation, and poetry 24
suppressed emotions 4–5, 7
Survivors' Poetry 117

tasks of mourning 63–4
therapy

goals and aspirations 77–9
in adolescence 24
in middle age 31–2, 34–5
making sense of life 74–6
poet's views 12–13
and spirituality 37–8, 39–43
and transitions 16
and unfinished business 68
and use of metaphors 74–6
see also poetry in therapy
Thomas, DM 4, 43–4
Thompson, K 144
Thompson, N 56
Thorne, B 38
The Thought Fox (Hughes) 8–9
time, spirituality and nature 48–9
training and creative writing
individual therapy 144
journal writing 144–6
personal development groups 144
poetry and creative writing 143–50
professional development 146–7
transactional analysis 76–7
transcribing poetry 135–6
transitions in life 15–16
adolescence 19–24
child birth and parenthood 27–31
see also stages of life
The Transpersonal (Rowan) 41
transpersonal therapy 41–2
Trower, P 82
trust, stages of life (Erikson) 18–19
The Truth is Optional (Carmichael) 123
Twelfth Night (Shakespeare) 7
Twelve Songs (Auden) 54–5, 66

Ulysses 73–4
unconscious, unexpressed feelings 4–5

'unfinished business' 68

vengeful thoughts 59

waiting rooms, and poetry projects 115
Walking Away – for Sean (Day Lewis)
30–1, 94
Warning (Joseph) 34
The Wasteland (Eliot) 10
We Real Cool (Brooks) 21–2
Welsh National Opera 121, 128–31
What Every Women Should Carry (Dooley)
101
What's on my Mind (Schneider) 111
Why I am angry that Ben is dead
(Hermione) 92
When I Have Fears (Keats) 47
Whitemore, D 41–2
Williams, H 17–18
Williamson, C 125
Windsor Declaration (1998) 107
Winnicott, D 7, 29
wisdom 73
WNO MAX (Welsh National Opera
educational department) 121
Wolberg, L 63
Wolf, V 10
Wood, S 139–40
Worden, W 63–4, 67
Wordsworth, W 17, 44, 46
workshops see poetry workshops
Wozzeck (Berg) 129–30
writing poetry see creative writing

Yalom, I 54, 81, 147
Yeats, WB 4, 59, 78, 133, 143
Your Face (Hill) 59

For Product Safety Concerns and Information please contact our EU
representative GPSR@taylorandfrancis.com
Taylor & Francis Verlag GmbH, Kaufingerstraße 24, 80331 München, Germany

www.ingramcontent.com/pod-product-compliance
Ingram Content Group UK Ltd.
Pitfield, Milton Keynes, MK11 3LW, UK
UKHW051829180425
457613UK00022B/1173